Prostate cancer
diet cookbook for newly diagnosed
2024

100 easy and healthy recipes to support your prostatic journey

BY

FRAZIER BOB

Table of contents

Introduction

Welcome to the Prostate Cancer Cookbook, a lovingly created culinary guide for anyone coping with a recent prostate cancer diagnosis. This cookbook is a handbook meant to support and empower those who are starting this journey, not just a list of recipes. In times of uncertainty, diet is essential for maintaining general health and controlling side effects of medication. These dishes are carefully chosen to offer tasty, nutrient-rich options that are in line with dietary guidelines for individuals receiving treatment, with an emphasis on prostate health. This cookbook attempts to transform the kitchen into a source of power and healing, with everything from prostate-friendly products to useful meal planning advice. Whether you're looking for solace, diversity, or just a means to improve your health via flavorful dishes, let this cookbook be your ally in fostering a balanced and enjoyable approach to nutrition during this pivotal time.

CHAPTER ONE

RECOGNIZING NUTRITION AND PROSTATE CANCER

The right Nutrition

Appropriate diet has a big impact on how people with prostate cancer feel about their health. A customized and well-balanced diet can be extremely important for improving general health, supporting the efficacy of treatment, and controlling symptoms. Sufficient consumption of micronutrients including fiber, omega-3 fatty acids, and antioxidants may be beneficial to prostate health. Fruits and vegetables that are high in antioxidants can help fight oxidative stress and lower the chance that prostate cancer will progress. A diet rich in fiber can also help maintain digestive health and help minimize the negative effects of some medications. Flaxseeds and fish, which are high in omega-3 fatty acids, may have advantageous anti-inflammatory effects.

Furthermore, as obesity is associated with an increased risk of developing aggressive prostate cancer, keeping a healthy weight through appropriate nutrition is crucial.

The Benefits of the right Nutrition:

Adopting a healthy diet can be extremely beneficial for people who have just received a prostate cancer diagnosis. Beyond the physical effects, during this difficult journey, a well-balanced diet customized to meet individual needs becomes essential for general wellbeing. Maintaining a strong immune system, promoting energy levels, and controlling treatment-related symptoms are all made possible by proper nutrition. It is essential for lowering inflammation and fostering the best possible prostate health by providing specific nutrients. Making thoughtful food choices also makes it easier to maintain a healthy weight, which improves treatment results. The psychological boost that comes from feeling in charge of one's health emphasizes how crucial it is to recognize the necessity of eating a healthy diet. Speaking with medical experts guarantees tailored advice, which makes nutrition an invaluable ally for people managing the intricacies of a newly diagnosed prostate cancer.

Phytochemicals and antioxidants

Antioxidants and phytochemicals are important for maintaining the health of people who have just received a prostate cancer diagnosis.
1. Phytochemicals: Lower Risk of Cancer Naturally occurring substances found in plant-based diets called phytochemicals have been linked to a decreased risk of prostate cancer. Eating a range of

fruits, vegetables, and whole grains yields a varied assortment of these advantageous substances.
 Anti-Inflammatory Properties: A variety of phytochemicals have anti-inflammatory qualities that may aid in lowering inflammation that is connected to the development of cancer.

2. Antioxidants: Cellular Defense: Rich in foods like berries, almonds, and leafy greens, antioxidants aid in shielding cells from harm brought on by free radicals. For those receiving treatment for prostate cancer, this protection is essential.
 DNA Repair: Antioxidants help to maintain healthy cells by assisting in DNA repair processes, which may also prevent the formation of cancerous cells. It can be advantageous to include a wide range of foods high in antioxidants and phytochemicals in the diet.

Hydration

 hydration is an essential ally. Beyond its benefits to general health, drinking enough water becomes extremely important at this difficult time. Maintaining adequate hydration supports kidney function, which may be influenced by specific medicines, and helps control typical side effects of therapy, such as nausea and exhaustion. Drinking water throughout the day helps reduce symptoms such as dry mouth, which makes treatments more comfortable.

Hydration is important for digestion and for promoting general health, especially for people adjusting to dietary changes or managing the gastrointestinal side effects of treatment. Though it's obvious how important it is to stay hydrated, everyone has different demands.

Minerals and Vital Vitamins

Minerals That Are Good for the Prostate:
* Selenium Selenium, which is well-known for its antioxidant qualities, is essential for preserving prostate health. It might lessen the chance of prostate cancer and provide protection against oxidative stress. Whole grains, salmon, and Brazil nuts are foods high in selenium.
* Zinc: Zinc affects prostate health and is necessary for immune system function. Prostate cancer risk is inversely correlated with adequate zinc levels. Lean meats, nuts, and dairy products are good dietary sources.
* Calcium: While consuming too much calcium may raise your chance of developing prostate cancer, it's still vital to keep your calcium levels in check for general health. Calcium-rich foods include leafy greens, dairy products, and fortified foods.
*Vitamin D is a crucial vitamin for prostate cancer. This vitamin may help lower the risk of prostate cancer and is essential for immune system function. Adequate levels are facilitated by sun exposure and meals high in vitamin D, such as

eggs, dairy products with added vitamin D, and
fatty fish.
*Egg: Vitamin E functions as an antioxidant,
preventing cellular damage. According to certain
research, vitamin E may help prevent prostate
cancer. Nuts, Leafy greens, and seeds are good
sources.
*Calcium: Vitamin C, which is well-known for its
antioxidant qualities, boosts immunity and might
lessen oxidative stress. strawberries, peppers, and
citrus fruits are great sources.

Keeping a balanced intake on macronutrient

During this difficult period, every
macronutrient—fats, proteins, and carbs—has a
unique function in promoting general health.
 Choosing complex carbs such as fruits,
vegetables, and whole grains gives you long-lasting
energy, which is important when you're trying to
fight off the weariness that comes with cancer and
its therapies. These foods also provide important
minerals and vitamins.
Sufficient consumption of protein is essential for
immune system and tissue repair, two aspects of
the body's defense against cancer. Good sources
of protein include fish, poultry, lentils, dairy
products, and lean meats.
 Selecting good fats promotes general health, such
as those in almonds, avocados, and olive oil. Fatty

fish, which are high in omega-3 fatty acids, can be advantageous because of their anti-inflammatory qualities.

Foods to reduce

* Processed Meats: Minimize intake of processed meats like sausages and hot dogs, as they may be associated with an increased risk of prostate cancer.
* High-Fat Dairy: Reduce consumption of high-fat dairy products, as excessive saturated fat intake may have links to prostate cancer progression.
* Saturated Fats: Cut back on saturated fats found in fried foods, certain oils, and fatty cuts of meat, as they may contribute to inflammation.
* Excessive Calcium:** While calcium is essential, avoid excessive intake, as it might be associated with an increased risk of prostate cancer. Moderate consumption of dairy and calcium-rich foods is advisable.
* Excessively Spicy Foods: For some individuals, very spicy foods can irritate the digestive system. Moderation in spicy food intake may be beneficial.
* Alcohol: Limit your alcohol intake because it may interfere with some therapies and has been associated with a higher risk of prostate cancer.
* Sugar-filled Foods and Drinks: Limit your use of sweetened beverages, desserts, and sugary snacks as these may aggravate inflammation and cause weight gain.

* Overindulgence in red meat: Limit your consumption of red and processed meats, even if lean protein is vital, as they may raise your risk of prostate cancer.

Nourishing foods to Embrace

1. Vegetables with Crucifers: Compounds found in kale, cauliflower, and broccoli may offer protection against prostate cancer.
2. Tomatoes: Tomatoes, being high in lycopene, are good for the prostate. When they are cooked, more lycopene is released for absorption.
3. Fatty Fish: Prostate health may benefit from the anti-inflammatory properties of salmon and trout, which are rich in omega-3 fatty acids.
4. Berries: Antioxidants from blueberries, strawberries, and raspberries promote general health.
5 Tea (Green Tea): Green tea, well-known for its antioxidant qualities, might be good for prostate health.
Whole Grains: Whole wheat, quinoa, and brown rice all offer sustaining energy along with vital nutrients.
7. Nuts and Seeds: Pumpkin seeds, walnuts, almonds, and flax seeds provide vital nutrients and healthy fats.
8. Legumes: Chickpeas, lentils, and beans are good sources of plant-based fiber and protein.
9. Slim Meat: To satisfy your protein needs while reducing your intake of saturated fat, use lean

meats like chicken or plant-based alternatives like tofu.

10. Vibrant Vegetables: Sweet potatoes, carrots, and bell peppers are rich in vitamins and minerals.

Building a balanced diet

Prioritize a colorful array of fruits and vegetables. These provide essential vitamins, minerals, and antioxidants crucial for immune support and overall well-being.

Choose lean protein sources such as fish, poultry, tofu, and legumes. Protein supports tissue repair and immune function, essential aspects during cancer treatment. Incorporate whole grains like brown rice, quinoa, and whole wheat, offering complex carbohydrates for sustained energy.

Add a source of healthy fats like avocados, nuts, seeds, and olive oil. Omega-3 fatty acids, found in fatty fish, can contribute to anti-inflammatory. BBe mindful of saturated fats, limiting red and processed meats, high-fat dairy, and certain oils to manage inflammation and support heart health.

CHAPTER TWO

ENERGY BOOSTERS
BREAKFAST

Frittata Muffins with Spinach and Feta:

Ingredients:
- Six big eggs
- Half a cup of milk (vegan or dairy)
- Half cup crumbled feta cheese
- One cup chopped fresh spinach
- 1/4 cup chopped red bell pepper
- 1/4 cup coarsely chopped red onion
- Season with salt and pepper
- Grease muffin tin with cooking spray or olive oil

Instructions:
- Put the oven on to 375°F, or 190°C. Use cooking spray or olive oil to grease a muffin pan.
- Whisk the eggs and milk together thoroughly in a bowl.
- Add sliced red bell pepper, finely chopped red onion, crumbled feta, and chopped spinach to the egg mixture.
- Put salt and pepper for seasoning.
- Evenly fill each cup in the muffin tin with the mixture, about two thirds full.

• Bake the frittata muffins for about 18 to 20 minutes, or until they are set and have a hint of color on top.
• After letting the muffins cool for a few minutes, carefully take them out of the muffin tray.
The savory taste of feta, the necessary nutrients from spinach, and the protein boost from the eggs all come together in these frittata muffins.

Turkey and Vegetable Breakfast Wrap:

Ingredients:
- One spinach or whole-grain wrap
Two to three thin slices of lean turkey breast; half a cup of mixed veggies, sautéed or grilled (spinach, bell peppers, onions)
- One spoonful of Greek yogurt or hummus to spread
- Optional fresh herbs, such as chives or parsley
To taste, add salt and pepper.

Instructions:
• Place the wrapper onto a dish or tidy surface.
• Cover the center of the wrap with a thin coating of Greek yogurt or hummus.
• Arrange the lean turkey breast slices on top of the mixture.
• Place the mixed vegetables, either grilled or sautéed, on top of the turkey pieces.
• Season with salt and pepper to taste and, if wanted, sprinkle with fresh herbs.

● To create a secure wrap, fold in the sides of the wrap and roll it up securely from the bottom.
This turkey breakfast wrap offers a good mix of lean protein, several vegetables for important nutrients, and fiber from the whole-grain wrap.

Oatmeal with Berries:

Ingredients:
- Half cup of traditional rolled oats
- One cup of water or plant-based or dairy milk
- An optional pinch of salt
- Half cup of mixed berries, including strawberries, raspberries, and blueberries
- One tablespoon of chopped nuts (walnuts, almonds) for healthy fats and texture
- One teaspoon (optional) of honey or maple syrup for sweetness
- Half a teaspoon of ground flaxseeds, if desired

Instructions:
● Bring the milk or water to a low boil in a saucepan.
● Add the rolled oats and, if preferred, a pinch of salt. Lower the heat to a simmer and cook the oats for around five minutes, stirring from time to time, or until they become creamy and the desired consistency.
● Take the saucepan off of the burner and give it a minute to thicken.

• Spoon the oats into a bowl, garnish with chopped nuts and mixed berries, and drizzle with maple syrup or honey, if preferred.
• You can optionally top with ground flaxseeds to offer even more nutritional value.
This breakfast offers antioxidants from the berries, fiber from the oats, and good fats from the nuts.

Vegetable and Tofu Scramble

Ingredients:
- Half a brick of crumbled firm tofu
- One cup of chopped mixed veggies, including bell peppers, cherry tomatoes, spinach, and mushrooms
- One-four cup coarsely sliced red onion - minced garlic clove
- One tablespoon of olive oil
- Half a teaspoon of powdered turmeric (for color)
- Season with salt and pepper
- Garnish with fresh herbs, such as parsley or chives, if desired

Instructions:
• In a pan over medium heat, warm the olive oil.
• Add the minced garlic and the finely sliced red onion. Onions should be sautéed until transparent.
• Place the mixed vegetables in the pan and heat them through just a little bit.
• To simulate the texture of scrambled eggs, crumble the firm tofu into the pan.

• Drizzle the tofu with turmeric powder for a golden color (and potential anti-inflammatory benefits).
• Add salt and pepper to taste and season the mixture. Make sure to thoroughly mix each component.
• Cook the tofu for a further five to seven minutes, or until it is thoroughly cooked and has absorbed the flavors of the veggies.
• If preferred, garnish with fresh herbs.
With a variety of vibrant vegetables, this Vegetable and Tofu Scramble offers a plant-based source of protein. Turmeric contributes a warm hue and possibly anti-inflammatory qualities.

Greek Yogurt Parfait with Nuts and Honey

Ingredients:
- One cup plain, low-fat, or non-fat Greek yogurt
- One-four cup chopped mixed nuts (walnuts and almonds).
- Half cup mixed berries (strawberries, raspberries, and blueberries)
- One tablespoon honey
- One-four cup ground flaxseeds (optional for increased omega-3 fatty acids and fiber)

Instructions:
• Place half of the Greek yogurt in the bottom of a serving glass or bowl.
• Sprinkle some mixed nuts on top of the yogurt.
• Spoon half of the honey onto the almonds.

• Spread the leftover Greek yogurt over another layer.

•Place the remaining honey and mixed berries over top.

 You can optionally add ground flaxseeds to the top for added nutritious value.

• Present right away and savor!

This Greek Yogurt Parfait has plenty of protein from the Greek yogurt, good fats from the nuts, and berries and honey for natural sweetness.

Mushroom and Tomato Breakfast Burrito

Ingredients:

- One spinach or whole-grain tortilla
- One cup sliced mushrooms
- One medium tomato chopped
- Two large beaten eggs
- One-four cup coarsely sliced red onion
- minced garlic clove
- One tablespoon of olive oil
- To taste, add salt and pepper
- Garnish with fresh herbs such as parsley or cilantro
- A serving of salsa or spicy sauce (optional)

Instructions:

• In a pan over medium heat, warm the olive oil.
• Add the minced garlic and the finely sliced red onion. Onions should be sautéed until transparent.

• When the mushrooms release their moisture and turn golden brown, add the sliced ones to the pan and simmer.
• Add the diced tomatoes to the pan and let them soften for a few minutes.
• Transfer the veggies to one side of the skillet and transfer the beaten eggs to the other.
• After the eggs are well cooked, scramble them and combine them with the tomato and mushroom mixture.
• Add salt and pepper to taste and season the mixture. Make sure to thoroughly mix each component.
• For a few seconds, reheat the tortilla in a dry pan or the microwave.
• Spoon the egg mixture with the mushrooms and tomato into the tortilla's middle.
• To create a burrito, fold the tortilla over the filling and garnish with fresh herbs if like.
• If desired, serve with hot sauce or salsa.
The eggs, mushrooms, and tomatoes in this breakfast burrito make it a high-protein choice.

Salmon and Cream Cheese Bagel

Ingredients:
- One whole-grain bagel
- Two ounces of cured salmon
- One tablespoon of drained capers
- Two tablespoons of cream cheese (light or standard)
- One-four thinly sliced red onion

- Fresh dill for garnish
- Serving wedges of lemon

Instructions:
• Toast the whole-grain bagel to your preferred texture by slicing it in half.
• Evenly distribute cream cheese over the bagel's two sides.
• Arrange smoked salmon pieces atop the cream cheese.
• To add a flavorful pop to the salmon, sprinkle it with capers.
• Top with finely sliced red onion.
• Add some fresh dill as a garnish for taste and freshness.
• For a zesty touch, serve with lemon slices on the side.
This salmon and cream cheese bagel has a lot of protein from the cream cheese and the salmon, as well as omega-3 fatty acids. It also tastes good because it has capers, red onion, and dill.

Whole Grain Toast with Avocado and Tomato Slices

Ingredients:
-A ripe avocado;
- Two slices of whole-grain bread
-One medium tomato, thinly sliced
-salt and pepper to taste;
-optional garnish of red pepper flakes or herbs

Instructions:
• Toast the slices of whole-grain bread as desired.
• Peel and pit the ripe avocado while the bread is browning.
• Using a fork, mash the avocado in a bowl until the consistency that you like is achieved.
• Evenly cover each piece of toast with mashed avocado.
• Place a few thin tomato slices over the avocado.
• Season the tomatoes with salt and pepper to taste.
• You can add more flavor by garnishing with your preferred herbs or red pepper flakes.

An option that is high in nutrients and beneficial to the prostate is this whole grain toast with avocado and tomato slices. Tomatoes contain antioxidants, and avocados offer good fats.

Sweet Potato Hash with Poached Eggs

Ingredients:
- One large sweet potato, chopped and skinned
- One tablespoon olive oil
- Half a diced red bell pepper
- Half a red onion, cut finely
- Two minced garlic cloves
-One tsp of paprika
- 4 big eggs
- Put Salt and pepper to taste
- Optional fresh parsley garnish

Instructions:

- In a big skillet over medium heat, warm up the olive oil.
- Add the chopped sweet potatoes to the skillet and toss occasionally while cooking until they are soft and golden brown.
- Mix the minced garlic, chopped red onion, and diced red bell pepper with the sweet potatoes. Cook the vegetables for a little longer until they are tender.
- Top the mixture with paprika, salt, and pepper. Mix thoroughly to blend.
- In the hash, make four wells and crack an egg into each.
- Put the skillet lid on and allow the eggs to poach for approximately five to seven minutes, or until the yolks are still runny but the whites are set.
- You can add some fresh parsley as a garnish once the eggs are cooked to your preference.
- Present the poached eggs and sweet potato hash right away.

It offers a good ratio of protein, healthy fats, and complex carbohydrates.

Fruit Salad with Greek Yogurt

Ingredients:
- One cup plain, low-fat, or non-fat Greek yogurt
- One cup of chopped mixed fruits (grapes, kiwis, melon, pineapple, and berries).
- One tablespoon of maple syrup or honey, if desired for sweetness

- One tablespoon of optionally chopped nuts
(walnuts, almonds) for crunch
- Optional fresh mint leaves as a garnish

Instructions:
• Place the Greek yogurt in a bowl and well mix in
the honey or maple syrup, if desired.
• Chop a range of fruits and mix them into the
yogurt-filled bowl.
• Gently mix the fruits to coat them thoroughly in
the yogurt.
• If preferred, top with chopped nuts for more
crunch.
• Add some fresh mint leaves as a garnish for a
refreshing touch.
Protein is provided by Greek yogurt; vitamins,
antioxidants, and natural sweetness are found in a
variety of fruits. Nuts offer texture and good fats.

Egg White Omelette with Spinach and Mushrooms

Ingredients:
- One cup of egg whites, or roughly eight big egg
whites
- Half cup sliced mushrooms
- One cup chopped fresh spinach
- One-four cup coarsely sliced red onion
- minced garlic clove
- One tablespoon of olive oil
- Season with salt and pepper

- Garnish with fresh herbs, such as parsley or chives, if desired
- Goat or Feta cheese for flavor enhancement (optional)

Instructions:
- In a nonstick skillet over medium heat, warm the olive oil.
- Add the minced garlic and the finely sliced red onion. Onions should be sautéed until transparent.
- Place the sliced mushrooms in the skillet and heat them through until they start to brown and release moisture.
- Cook the spinach in the skillet with chopped leaves until it wilts.
- Beat the egg whites until foamy in a bowl. Over the vegetables in the skillet, pour the egg whites.
- Permit the egg whites to firm up on the sides. Using a spatula, gently lift the edges to allow the raw egg to run below.
- Using the spatula, fold the omelette in half once the egg whites are mostly set.
- Add salt and pepper to taste If preferred, garnish with crumbled goat cheese or feta and fresh herbs. The mushrooms and spinach provide minerals and vitamins, making this tasty and nutritious.

Chia Seed Pudding with Berries

Ingredients:
-One-fourth cup chia seeds

- One cup of almond milk, unsweetened (or any choice milk)
- One tablespoon of maple syrup or honey, if desired for sweetness
- Half a teaspoon of essence from vanilla
- A mixture of berries (strawberries, raspberries, and blueberries) as a topping - Chopped or sliced almonds as an optional garnish

Instructions:
• Place the chia seeds, almond milk, vanilla essence, honey (or maple syrup,
if desired), and a bowl. Blend thoroughly.
• To prevent clumping, whisk the mixture once more after letting it sit for about five minutes.
• To enable the chia seeds to absorb the liquid and take on the consistency of pudding, cover the bowl and place it in the refrigerator for at least two hours or overnight.
• Give the chia pudding a good swirl before serving.
• Transfer the chia pudding into dishes or glasses for serving.
• Add a layer of mixed berries on top, and if like, decorate with chopped or sliced almonds.
• Present cold and savor!
Berries offer antioxidants and a naturally sweet taste, while chia seeds offer fiber and omega-3 fatty acids.

Blueberry and Walnut Overnight Oats

Ingredients:
- Half cup plain, fat-free, or low-fat Greek yogurt
- Half cup old-fashioned rolled oats
- Half cup almond milk, without sugar added (or any favorite milk)
- Half cup frozen or fresh blueberries
- Two tablespoons of walnuts, chopped
- One tablespoon of maple syrup or honey, if desired for sweetness
- Half a teaspoon of essence from vanilla

Instructions:
• Put the rolled oats, Greek yogurt, almond milk, chopped walnuts, blueberries, and vanilla extract (or honey, if desired) in a jar or other lidded container.
• Make sure all components are fully combined by giving it a good stir.
• To help the oats absorb the liquid and soften, cover the jar or container with a lid and chill it for at least four hours or overnight.
• Give the overnight oats a nice toss before serving.
• For added crunch and freshness, you can add chopped walnuts and more blueberries on top, if you'd like.
• You may eat the Walnut and Blueberry Overnight Oats right out of the jar or you can transfer them to a bowl.

This recipe for overnight oats is a quick and wholesome breakfast choice. Antioxidants are provided by blueberries, and omega-3 fatty acids and a delightful crunch are added by walnuts.

Cottage Cheese with Pineapple Chunks

Ingredients:
- One cup of cottage cheese, regular or low-fat
- Half a cup of fresh chunk pineapple
- One tablespoon of chopped nuts (walnuts, almonds) for texture addition (optional)
- Optional fresh mint leaves as a garnish
- Maple syrup or honey to drizzle (optional)

Instructions:
- Put the Scoop cottage cheese into a bowl.
- Mix the cottage cheese with chunks of fresh pineapple.
- For extra texture, if preferred, top with chopped nuts.
- For an added touch of sweetness, you can optionally pour some honey or maple syrup over the mixture.
- If preferred, garnish with fresh mint leaves.
- Enjoy the ingredients as layers or gently combine them together.

Protein and calcium are provided by cottage cheese, while natural sweetness and vitamins are added by pineapple.

Whole Grain Waffles with Nut Butter and Banana Slices

Ingredients:
- Two whole grain waffles (homemade or from the supermarket)
- Two tablespoons of nut butter (peanut or almond).
- Slice one medium banana
- For extra crunch, add 1 tablespoon of chopped nuts (almonds or walnuts, optional).
- Maple syrup or honey to drizzle (optional)

Instructions:
- Toast the whole grain waffles as directed on the package, or to the desired degree of crispness.
- Cover each waffle with a thick layer of nut butter.
- Place slices of banana over the layer of nut butter.
- To add more texture to the bananas, feel free to sprinkle chopped nuts on top.
- You may optionally add a little sweetness to the waffles by drizzling them with honey or maple syrup.
6• Present the Whole Grain Waffles along with Banana Slices right away.

This breakfast choice includes bananas for natural sweetness and potassium, nut butter for healthy fats and protein, and whole grains for fiber.

ENERGY BOOSTER SMOOTHIES

Chocolate Avocado Indulgence

Ingredients:
- Half a ripe avocado
- One tablespoon of powder unsweetened cocoa
- One tiny banana
- One scoop of chocolate protein powder with flavoring (optional)
- One cup almond milk (or your favorite type of milk)
- One tablespoon of almond butter
- Ice cubes, if desired
- For sweetness, honey or maple syrup (optional)

Instructions:
- Remove the ripe avocado's pit.
- Put the avocado, banana, cocoa powder, almond milk, almond butter, and protein powder (if using) in a blender.
- Blend until creamy and smooth. If you want your consistency cooler, add some ice cubes.
- After tasting the smoothie, if you would like it sweeter, add more honey or maple syrup.
- Blend one more to include any additional sugar. This smoothie combines the creamy smoothness and beneficial fat of avocado with the rich chocolate flavor of cocoa powder. The banana provides natural sweetness, and the almond butter adds even more richness.

Protein Berry Boost smoothie

Ingredients:
- One cup of mixed berries, including raspberries, strawberries, and blueberries
- One scoop of mixed berries or vanilla-flavored protein powder
- One tablespoon of chia seeds or almond butter for extra protein and good fats
- One cup almond milk (or your favorite type of milk)
- Ice cubes, if desired
- For sweetness, honey or maple syrup (optional)

Instructions:
• Put the mixed berries, almond milk, protein powder, and chia seeds or almond butter in a blender.
• Add some ice cubes to the blender if you'd like it cooler.
• Blend until thoroughly mixed and smooth.
• After tasting the smoothie, if you would like it sweeter, add more honey or maple syrup.
• Blend one more to include any additional sugar.
• Transfer into a glass and savor your Berry Protein Boost!
The protein powder, almond butter, or chia seeds in this smoothie give it an extra protein boost while the mixed berries are a great source of antioxidants.

Almond Joy Delight smoothie

Ingredients:
- Half a ripe banana
- One tablespoon of almond butter
- One tablespoon of unsweetened shredded coconut
- One tablespoon of almonds, chopped
- One tablespoon of unsweetened cocoa powder
- One cup coconut milk (or your favorite kind of milk)
- Ice cubes, if desired
- For sweetness, honey or maple syrup (optional)

Instructions:
- Cut the ripe banana into slices.
- Put the banana slices, chopped almonds, shredded coconut, almond butter, cocoa powder, and coconut milk in a blender.
- Include some ice cubes in the blender if you'd like it cooler.
- Blend until creamy and smooth.
- If you would want the smoothie to be sweeter, taste it and add more honey or maple syrup.
- Blend one more to include any additional sugar. Rich tastes of cocoa, coconut, and almonds come together in this smoothie to create a delightful and filling treat. Protein and good fats are added by the chopped almonds and almond butter.

Detoxifying Green Apple Smoothie

Ingredients:
- One cup coconut water (or your choice liquid)
- Half cucumber, peeled and sliced
- A handful of spinach leaves
- Half lemon, juiced
- Ice cubes, if desired
- Optional fresh mint leaves as a garnish
- For sweetness, honey or maple syrup (optional)

Instructions:
- Cut the green apple into pieces.
- Chop the cucumber and peel it.
- Put the cut cucumber, spinach leaves, green apple, lemon juice, and coconut water in a blender.
- You can add ice cubes to the blender if you'd like it colder.
- Blend until thoroughly mixed and smooth.
- If you would want the smoothie to be sweeter, taste it and add more honey or maple syrup.
- Blend one more to include any additional sugar. Green apple, cucumber, and spinach are just a few of the detoxifying components found in this cool smoothie. The coconut water keeps you hydrated while the lemon gives it a zesty bite.

Tropical Paradise Energizer smoothie

Ingredients:
- Half a cup of chopped pineapple
- Half cup chunky mango
- One-half half banana

-A handful of leaves from spinach
- Half cup plain, low-fat, or non-fat Greek yogurt
- One-third cup chia seeds
- One cup of coconut water, or any other desired beverage
- Ice cubes, if desired
- Optional fresh mint leaves as a garnish
- For sweetness, honey or maple syrup (optional)

Instructions:
• Put the banana, spinach leaves, Greek yogurt, chia seeds, pineapple and mango pieces, and coconut water in a blender.
• Add some ice cubes to the blender if you'd like it cooler.
• Blend until thoroughly mixed and smooth.
• After tasting the smoothie, if you would like it sweeter, add more honey or maple syrup.
• Blend one more to include any additional sugar. The pineapple, mango, and spinach in this tropical smoothie are packed with vitamins, minerals, and antioxidants. Protein is added by the Greek yogurt, and fiber and good fats are provided by the chia seeds.

Kiwi Coconut Dream

Ingredients:
- Two sliced and peeled kiwis
- Half a cup of coconut milk
- Half a cup of spinach leaves
- One half banana

- One-third cup chia seeds
- Ice cubes, if desired
- Optional fresh coconut slices as a garnish
- For sweetness, honey or maple syrup (optional)

Instructions:
- First, peel and cut the kiwis.
- Put the banana, chia seeds, spinach leaves, coconut milk, and sliced kiwis in a blender.
- Include some ice cubes in the blender if you'd like it cooler.
- Blend until thoroughly mixed and smooth.
- If you would want the smoothie to be sweeter, taste it and add more honey or maple syrup.
- Blend one more to include any additional sugar.

Pear Ginger Zinger smoothie

Ingredients:
- One ripe pear, cored and diced
- Half an inch of fresh ginger, peeled and grated
- Half a cup of plain non-fat, or low-fat Greek yogurt
- One tablespoon of chia seeds
- One cup of almond milk (or your favorite beverage)
- Ice cubes, if desired
- Optional fresh mint leaves as a garnish
- For sweetness, honey or maple syrup (optional)

Instructions:
- Cut the ripe pear into pieces.
- Grate and peel the raw ginger.

• Put the chopped pear, almond milk, Greek yogurt, chia seeds, and grated ginger in a blender.
• You can add ice cubes to the blender if you'd like it colder.
• Blend until thoroughly mixed and smooth.
• If you would want the smoothie to be sweeter, taste it and add more honey or maple syrup.
• Blend one more to include any additional sugar.

Blueberry Walnut Wonder smoothie

Ingredients:
half a cup of frozen or fresh blueberries
- One-fourth cup of walnuts
- One -half banana
- Half cup plain, low-fat, or non-fat Greek yogurt
- One cup almond milk, or any other preferred beverage
- Ice cubes, if desired
- For sweetness, honey or maple syrup (optional)

Instructions:
• Put the banana, Greek yogurt, almond milk, walnuts, and blueberries in a blender.
• Add some ice cubes to the blender if you'd like it cooler.
• Blend until thoroughly mixed and smooth.
• After tasting the smoothie, if you would like it sweeter, add more honey or maple syrup.
• Blend one more to include any additional sugar.

Chia Berry Antioxidant Bowl

Ingredients:
- Half a cup of chia seeds
- Half cup of mixed berries, including raspberries, strawberries, and blueberries
- Half cup plain, low-fat, or non-fat Greek yogurt
- One-fourth cup of granola
- One tablespoon (optional) of honey or maple syrup for sweetness
- Optional fresh mint leaves as a garnish

Instructions:
- Put the chia seeds and half a cup of water in a basin. Give it a good stir, then leave it for at least fifteen minutes, or until the chia seeds start to gel.
- Arrange the chia seeds in a layer at the base of a serving bowl when they have thickened.
- Transfer Greek yogurt onto the layer of chia seeds.
- Top the Greek yogurt with a mixture of berries.
- To add more crunch, scatter granola over the berries.
- Drizzle the bowl with honey or maple syrup, if preferred.
- Garnish with fresh mint leaves for a burst of freshness.

Green Powerhouse Smoothie

Ingredients:
- One cup of spinach leaves
- Half sliced and peeled cucumber

- Half cored and diced green apple
- Half pitted and peeled avocado
- Half lemon juiced
- One cup coconut water (or favorite drink)
- Ice cubes, if desired
- Optional fresh mint leaves as a garnish
- For sweetness, honey or maple syrup (optional)

Instructions:
• Put the spinach leaves, cucumber slices, avocado, diced green apple, lemon juice, and coconut water in a blender.
• Add some ice cubes to the blender if you'd like it cooler.
• Blend until thoroughly mixed and smooth.
• After tasting the smoothie, if you would like it sweeter, add more honey or maple syrup.
• Blend one more to include any additional sugar.

Mango Avocado Delight smoothie

Ingredients:
- Half a ripe mango, chopped and skinned - Half an avocado, pitted and peeled
- Half a banana
- Half cup plain, low-fat, or non-fat Greek yogurt
- One cup almond milk, or any other preferred milk
- Ice cubes, if desired
- Optional fresh mint leaves as a garnish
- For sweetness, honey or maple syrup (optional)

Instructions:
• Put the diced mango, avocado, banana, Greek yogurt, and almond milk in a blender.
• Add some ice cubes to the blender if you'd like it cooler.
• Blend until thoroughly mixed and smooth.
• After tasting the smoothie, if you would like it sweeter, add more honey or maple syrup.
• Blend one more to include any additional sugar.
• Transfer the contents into a glass, add some fresh mint leaves for decoration, and savor your Mango Avocado Delight!

Pineapple Mint Cooler

Ingredients:
- One cup of chunky pineapple
Scoop of fresh mint leaves
- Half a cucumber, cut into half and peeled
- Juiced half a lime
- One cup of coconut water (or any other chosen liquid)
- Half a teaspoon of freshly grated ginger
- Ice cubes, if desired
- For sweetness, honey or maple syrup (optional)

Instructions:
• Place the sliced cucumber, grated fresh ginger, lime juice, pineapple chunks, and fresh mint leaves in a blender with coconut water.
• Add some ice cubes to the blender if you'd like it cooler.

- Blend until thoroughly mixed and smooth.
- Taste the cooler, and if you want it sweeter, add more honey or maple syrup.
- Blend one more to include any additional sugar.
- Transfer the mixture into a glass, add a mint leaf as a garnish, and savor your Pineapple Mint Cooler!

Golden Turmeric Smoothie

Ingredients:
- Half cup chunky mango
- Half teaspoon of raw ginger, grated;
- Half teaspoon of crushed turmeric;
- Half banana
- Half cup plain, low-fat, or non-fat Greek yogurt
- A cup of coconut milk, or any other favored beverage
- Ice cubes, if desired
- Black pepper, optional, to improve the absorption of turmeric
- For sweetness, honey or maple syrup (optional)

Instructions:
- Put the banana, Greek yogurt, coconut milk, grated fresh ginger, crushed turmeric, and mango chunks into a blender.
- Add some ice cubes to the blender if you'd like it cooler.
- If preferred, add a small sprinkle of black pepper to help the turmeric absorb better.
- Blend until thoroughly mixed and smooth.

• If you would want the smoothie to be sweeter, taste it and add more honey or maple syrup.
• Blend once more to incorporate any added sweetener.

Berry Blast Smoothie

Ingredients:
- Half cup frozen or fresh blueberries
- Half cup of hulled strawberries
- One-half cup raspberries
- One half banana
- Half cup plain, low-fat, or non-fat Greek yogurt
- One cup almond milk, or any other preferred beverage
- Ice cubes, if desired
- For sweetness, honey or maple syrup (optional)

Instructions:
1. Place the banana, Greek yogurt, almond milk, blueberries, strawberries, and raspberries in a blender.
2. Add some ice cubes to the blender if you'd like it cooler.
3. Blend until thoroughly mixed and smooth.
4. After tasting the smoothie, if you would like it sweeter, add more honey or maple syrup.
5. Blend one more to include any additional sugar.

Antioxidant Citrus Smoothie

Ingredients:
- One orange, divided and peeled

- Half cup of mixed berries, including raspberries, strawberries, and blueberries
- One half banana
- Half cup plain, low-fat, or non-fat Greek yogurt
- Half a cup of coconut water
- Ice cubes, if desired
- Optional fresh mint leaves as a garnish
- For sweetness, honey or maple syrup (optional)

Instructions:
• Put the banana, Greek yogurt, coconut water, orange segments, and mixed berries in a blender.
• Add some ice cubes to the blender if you'd like it cooler.
• Blend until thoroughly mixed and smooth.
• After tasting the smoothie, if you would like it sweeter, add more honey or maple syrup.
• Blend one more to include any additional sugar.
• Transfer to a glass and top with a few fresh mint leaves.

Protein-Packed Almond Butter Smoothie

Ingredients:
- One banana
- One tablespoon of almond butter
- One scoop of chocolate or vanilla-flavored protein powder
- One cup almond milk, or any other preferred beverage
- Ice cubes, if desired

- One-half teaspoon of optional cinnamon
- For sweetness, honey or maple syrup (optional)

Instructions
• Put the banana, almond butter, protein powder, almond milk, and, if preferred, ice cubes in a blender.
• If you would like more flavor, add cinnamon.
• Blend until thoroughly mixed and smooth.
• After tasting the smoothie, if you would like it sweeter, add more honey or maple syrup.
• Blend one more to include any additional sugar.

Cherry Almond Bliss smoothie

Ingredients:
- Half cup pitted cherries, either fresh or frozen
- One tablespoon of almond butter
- One half banana
- One cup almond milk, or any other preferred beverage
- Ice cubes, if desired
- One-half teaspoon (optional) vanilla extract
- For sweetness, honey or maple syrup (optional)

Instructions:
• Put the cherries, almond butter, banana, almond milk, and ice cubes (if using) in a blender.
• If preferred, add vanilla extract for more taste.
• Blend until thoroughly mixed and smooth.
• After tasting the smoothie, if you would like it sweeter, add more honey or maple syrup.

• Blend one more to include any additional sugar.
The nutty richness of almond butter blends well
with the sweet and tangy flavors of cherries in this
smoothie.

Prostate Health Elixir smoothie

Ingredients:
- One-fourth cup pepitas, or pumpkin seeds
- Half cup of mixed berries, including raspberries,
strawberries, and blueberries
- One-half banana
- One spoonful of flaxseed meal
- One cup almond milk, or any other preferred
beverage
- Ice cubes, if desired
- Half a teaspoon of powdered turmeric
- For sweetness, honey or maple syrup (optional)

Instructions:
• Place the banana, ground flaxseeds, mixed
berries, pumpkin seeds, almond milk, and ice
cubes (if preferred) in a blender.
• Include the powdered turmeric, which has
anti-inflammatory qualities.
• Blend until thoroughly mixed and smooth.
• After tasting the smoothie, if you would like it
sweeter, add more honey or maple syrup.
• Blend one more to include any additional sugar.
Ingredients in this smoothie are recognized for their
possible advantages in supporting prostate health.

Carrot Cake Bliss smoothie

Ingredients:
- Half cup of carrots, shredded
- Half banana
- One-fourth cup of walnuts
-One-third cup chia seeds
- Half a teaspoon of ground cinnamon
- One cup almond milk, or any other preferred beverage
- Ice cubes, if desired
- For sweetness, honey or maple syrup (optional)

Instructions:
• Put the banana, shredded carrots, chia seeds, walnuts, ground cinnamon, almond milk, and ice cubes (if preferred) in a blender.
• Blend until thoroughly mixed and smooth.
• After tasting the smoothie, if you would like it sweeter, add more honey or maple syrup.
• Blend one more to include any additional sugar.
• Transfer into a glass and savor your blissful carrot cake!

CHAPTER THREE

MOUTH WATERING LUNCH

Spinach and Berry Salad with Chicken

Ingredients:
- One cup of mixed berries (strawberries, blueberries, and raspberries)
- Two cups of fresh spinach leaves
- One sliced grilled chicken breast
- 1/4 cup grated feta cheese (optional)
- 1/4 cup chopped walnuts
- A handmade balsamic vinaigrette dressing, which allows for greater control over the ingredients.
-To taste, add salt and pepper.

Instructions:
◇ Clean the fresh spinach leaves and pat dry. Put them in a big salad bowl.

◇ Divide the mixed berries among the spinach leaves. Place the grilled chicken slices on top of the grill.

◇ If you'd like, top the salad with crumbled feta cheese for a creamy texture and extra taste.

◇ Add some chopped walnuts to the salad to give it a delicious crunch and some good fats.

◇ Pour the salad with a balsamic vinaigrette dressing. Adjust the quantity to suit your tastes.

◇ A little pepper and salt can bring out the taste. Make adjustments based on personal preference.

◇ Gently toss the salad to make sure all of the ingredients are evenly distributed and dressed.

Whole Grain Couscous with Chickpeas

Ingredients:
- One cup of whole grain couscous
- One can (15 oz) of rinsed and drained chickpeas
- One cup of split cherry tomatoes
- Half diced cucumber
- One-fourth cup of finely chopped red onion
- One-fourth cup of chopped fresh parsley
- Two tablespoons olive oil
- One tablespoon lemon juice
- One teaspoon of ground cumin
- To taste, add salt and pepper

Instructions:
◇ Follow the cooking directions on the package for the whole grain couscous. Using a fork, fluff the cooked couscous and let it come to room temperature.

◇ Place the rinsed and drained chickpeas and cooked couscous in a large mixing basin.

◇ Stir into the couscous and chickpea mixture the diced cucumber, finely chopped red onion, split cherry tomatoes, and fresh parsley.

◇ To make the dressing, combine the olive oil, lemon juice, ground cumin, salt, and pepper in a small bowl.

◇ Over the couscous and chickpea mixture, drizzle the dressing. Make sure that every ingredient has an even coat.

◇ Gently toss the salad to spread the dressing and mix the ingredients.

◇ Tailor the amount of salt and pepper to your personal taste.

Caprese Salad with Grilled Chicken

Ingredients:
- Two skin-and bone-free chicken breasts
- Two large tomatoes, cut
- Two tablespoons olive oil
- Salt and pepper to taste
- One freshly sliced ball of mozzarella cheese
- New basil leaves
- Drizzling balsamic glaze

Instructions:

◇ Set the grill's temperature to medium-high.

◇ Season the chicken breasts with salt and pepper after rubbing them with olive oil.

◇ The chicken should be cooked through after 6 to 8 minutes on each side of the grill. Make sure the inside temperature reaches 74°C, or 165°F.

◇ After cooking, let the chicken rest for a few minutes before slicing.

◇ Arrange the grilled chicken, fresh mozzarella, and tomato slices on a serving plate.

◇ To enhance the taste, nestle fresh basil leaves in between the slices of mozzarella and tomato.

◇ Pour balsamic glaze over the salad. Use according to personal preference, either more or less.

◇ Sprinkle a small amount of salt and pepper on top of the constructed salad.

Turkey and Vegetable Skewers

Ingredients:
- One pound of cubed turkey breast
- One slice of zucchini
- One chopped red bell pepper
- One chopped yellow bell pepper

- One red onion, thinly sliced
- Cherry tomatoes
- Two tsp olive oil
- Two minced garlic cloves
- One teaspoon of oregano, dried
- Wooden skewers soaked in water for at least half an hour
- Salt and pepper to taste

Instructions:

◇ Set the grill's temperature to medium-high.

◇ Turkey cubes, olive oil, minced garlic, dried oregano, salt, and pepper should all be combined in a bowl. Give it at least fifteen minutes to marinate.

◇ On the wet wooden skewers, alternately thread the marinated turkey cubes, zucchini slices, bell pepper chunks, onion wedges, and cherry tomatoes.

◇ Arrange the skewers on the grill that have been preheated.

◇ Grill, rotating periodically, for about 8 to 10 minutes, or until the veggies are soft and the turkey is cooked through.

Broccoli and Chicken Alfredo

Ingredients:

- Eight ounces of whole-grain fettuccine pasta to add extra fiber.
- One tablespoon of olive oil
- One pound of boneless and stainless chicken breast, sliced into small pieces
- Two cups of broccoli florets
- Salt and pepper to taste
- Two minced garlic cloves
- One cup fat or low-fat-without Alfredo sauce
- Grated Parmesan cheese, half a cup
- Optional fresh parsley garnish

Instructions:
◇ Follow the directions on the package to cook the fettuccine pasta. After draining, set away.

◇ Heat olive oil in a big skillet over medium heat.
◇ After adding salt and pepper to the chicken pieces, sauté them until they are cooked through and have a light brown color. Bring out and place aside from the skillet.

◇ Place the broccoli florets and a little water in the same skillet. Steam the broccoli for several minutes with a cover on, until it becomes soft but retains its color.

◇ Add minced garlic to skillet and cook for approximately one minute.
◇ Put the Alfredo sauce and mix together.

◇ Add the broccoli, Alfredo sauce, and cooked chicken back to the skillet.

◇ Gently stir in the grated cheese, letting it melt into the sauce.

◇ Fill the skillet with the cooked fettuccine pasta. Mix everything together until the Alfredo sauce is evenly distributed throughout the spaghetti.

Vegetable and Brown Rice Bowl

Ingredients:
- One cup of brown rice, boiled as directed on the package
- One medium zucchini, sliced
- One tablespoon olive oil
- One bell pepper, cut into any hue
– One cup florets of broccoli
- One chopped or julienned carrot
- One cup of blanched snap peas
- Two chopped garlic cloves
- two teaspoons of soy sauce decreased in sodium
- One tablespoon of rice vinegar
- One teaspoon of optional sesame oil
- Optional sesame seeds as a garnish
- Chop green onions used as a garnish (optional)

Instructions:
◇ Follow the directions on the package to prepare the brown rice. Put aside.

◇ Heat olive oil in a big skillet or wok over medium-high heat.

◇ Snap peas, bell pepper, broccoli florets, julienned carrot, and zucchini slices should all be added to the skillet.

◇ The vegetables should be sautéed for 5 to 7 minutes, or until they are crisp-tender.

◇ Cook the veggies for a further one to two minutes, or until the garlic is aromatic, after adding the minced garlic.

◇ Combine soy sauce, rice vinegar, and sesame oil (if using) in a small bowl.

◇ Fill the skillet with the sautéed vegetables and add the prepared brown rice.

◇ Drizzle the rice and veggies with the prepared sauce. Mix everything together until thoroughly hot and properly mixed.

◇ If you'd like, garnish the Brown Rice and Vegetable Bowl with chopped green onions and sesame seeds.

Roasted Vegetable and Quinoa Stuffed Peppers

Ingredients:
-Four large bell peppers, cut in half and seeded;
- one cup of cooked quinoa, as directed on the box

- Two cups chopped mixed veggies (e.g., eggplant, zucchini, cherry tomatoes, red onion)
- Two tsp olive oil
- Two minced garlic cloves
- One teaspoon of oregano, dried
- One cup tomato sauce
- Salt and pepper to taste
- Half cup grated feta cheese (optional)
- Optional fresh parsley garnish

Instructions:

◇ Set the oven's temperature to 375°F, or 190°C.

◇ Halve the bell peppers and remove the seeds and membranes. Put them inside a dish for baking.

◇ Prepare the quinoa per the directions on the package. Put aside.

◇ Combine the chopped mixed veggies, minced garlic, dried oregano, olive oil, salt, and pepper in a bowl. Arrange the veggies onto a baking sheet and bake in the oven that has been preheated for 15 to 20 minutes, or until they become soft.

◇ Combine the cooked quinoa and roasted vegetables in a big bowl. Blend thoroughly.

◇ Divide the veggie combination and quinoa into each half of a bell pepper.

◇ Cover the filled peppers with tomato sauce.

◇ Bake the baking dish in the oven for about 25 to 30 minutes, or until the peppers are soft, covered with foil.

◇ In the final five minutes of baking, top the filled peppers with crumbled feta cheese, if desired.

Salmon and Quinoa Patties
Ingredients:
- One can (14 oz) of drained and flaked pink salmon
- One cup of cooked and cooled quinoa
- One-fourth cup of finely chopped red onion
- One-fourth cup of finely chopped bell pepper (any color)
- Two minced garlic cloves
- One-fourth cup finely chopped fresh parsley
- One-fourth cup whole wheat breadcrumbs
- One large egg
- One teaspoon Dijon mustard
-Taste-tested salt and pepper;
-Two teaspoons of olive oil for cooking

Instructions:
◇ Make sure the salmon in the can is drained and flaked. As directed on the package, prepare the quinoa and allow it to cool.

◇ The flaked salmon, cooked quinoa, minced garlic, diced bell pepper, chopped red onion, chopped parsley, Dijon mustard, egg, breadcrumbs, salt, and pepper should all be combined in a big bowl. Blend thoroughly.

◇ Create equal parts of the mixture and pat them into the desired form.

◇ In a skillet heat olive oil over medium heat.
◇ The salmon and quinoa patties should be cooked through and golden brown after 3 to 4 minutes on each side.

◇ After the patties are done, move them to a serving platter.

◇ If preferred, garnish with more fresh parsley.

Grilled Salmon Salad

Ingredients:
- One tablespoon olive oil
- Two salmon filets
- Mixed salad greens (e.g., spinach, arugula, romaine)
- Salt and pepper to taste
- Halved cherry tomatoes
- Sliced cucumber
- Thinly sliced red onion
- Sliced avocado
- Sliced lemons for garnishing

Instructions:

◇ One tablespoon each of balsamic vinegar and olive oil
◇ One teaspoon each of Dijon mustard
◇ To taste, salt and pepper
◇ Set your grill's temperature to medium-high.

◇ Season the salmon filets with salt and pepper after rubbing them with olive oil.

◇ Cook the salmon filets on the grill for 3 to 4 minutes on each side, or until they are thoroughly done. At 145°F (63°C), the inside temperature should be reached.

◇ After the salmon has finished cooking, let it sit for a few minutes before breaking it into small pieces.

◇ Put the mixed greens, cherry tomatoes, cucumber slices, red onion slices, and avocado in a big salad dish.

◇ To make the dressing, combine olive oil, balsamic vinegar, Dijon mustard, salt, and pepper in a small bowl.

◇ Top the salad with the flakes grilled salmon.

◇ Pour the salad and salmon with the dressing. Gently toss to mix.

Sweet Potato and Chickpea Salad

Ingredients:
- One can (15 oz) of drained and rinsed chickpeas;
- two medium sweet potatoes, peeled and diced;
-two tablespoons olive oil;
-one teaspoon each of ground cumin and paprika;
-To taste, add salt and pepper.
- Mixed salad greens, such as kale, spinach, and arugula
- Halved cherry tomatoes
- slice red onion thinly and Crumble Feta cheese if desired
-Dressing with balsamic vinaigrette

Instructions:
◇ Set the oven's temperature to 400°F, or 200°C.

◇ Combine the diced sweet potatoes and chickpeas with olive oil, paprika, ground cumin, salt, and pepper in a bowl. After placing them in a single layer on a baking sheet, roast them for 25 to 30 minutes, or until the chickpeas are crispy and the sweet potatoes are soft.

◇ Combine the cherry tomatoes, thinly sliced red onion, and mixed salad greens in a large salad dish.
◇ After roasting, incorporate the chickpeas and sweet potatoes into the salad bowl.

◇ You may add extra richness to the salad by sprinkling crumbled feta cheese on top.

◇ Pour the salad with a balsamic vinaigrette dressing. Gently toss to mix.

Egg Salad Lettuce Wraps

Ingredients:
- Four hard-boiled eggs, peeled and chopped;
- two tablespoons mayonnaise (you can instead use Greek or low-fat yogurt in place of the mayonnaise).
- One-fourth cup finely chopped celery
- Two tablespoons finely chopped red onion
- One teaspoon Dijon mustard
- Salt and pepper to taste
- Butter lettuce leaves (or your chosen lettuce kind)

Optional Ingredients:
- Dill, finely chopped
- Chopped chives - Sprouts
- Slices of avocado

Instructions:
◇ In a bowl, mix together the hard-boiled eggs, finely chopped celery, red onion, mayonnaise, Dijon mustard, and salt and pepper.

◇ Ensure that all of the ingredients are thoroughly mixed to create an even egg salad.

◇ Spoon a portion of the egg salad onto each lettuce leaf.

◇ Add optional ingredients like chopped dill, chopped chives, sprouts, or avocado slices on top of the egg salad.

◇ Fold the lettuce leaves to create wraps, enclosing the egg salad and optional add-ins.

Turkey and Avocado Wrap

Ingredients:
- One whole-wheat or whole-grain wrap
- A 4-oz turkey breast, cut
- Half of an avocado, cut
- One-fourth cup finely sliced cucumber
- One cup of halved cherry tomatoes
- Half a spoonful of hummus
- Fresh spinach or Romaine lettuce leaves
-To taste, add salt and pepper.

(Optional)
- Thinly chopped red onion
- Sprouts
- Mustard dijon

Instructions:
◇ Arrange the sliced turkey, avocado, cucumber, cherry tomatoes, hummus, and lettuce on the whole-grain wrap.

◇ Evenly spread the hummus in the center of the wrapper, around the edges with extra.

◇ Arrange the sliced turkey, avocado, cucumber, cherry tomatoes, and fresh lettuce leaves on top of the hummus.

◇ Toss to coat with a pinch of salt and pepper.

◇ For added taste, you can optionally add thinly sliced red onion, sprouts, or a splash of Dijon mustard.

◇ To make a secure wrap, fold in the sides of the wrap and then roll it up securely from the bottom.

Tuna Salad Lettuce Wraps
Ingredients:
- Two drained cans (5 ounces each) of tuna in water
- One-fourth cup finely sliced red onion
- One-fourth cup finely chopped celery
- One-fourth cup shredded carrot
- Two tablespoons mayonnaise (you may also use Greek or low-fat yogurt in place of this).
- One teaspoon Dijon mustard;
- Toppings of salt and pepper;
- Leaves of butter lettuce (or your favorite type of lettuce)
- Halved cherry tomatoes
- Slices of avocado
- Slices of cucumber

- Chopped fresh parsley

Instructions:
◇ In a bowl, mix together the drained tuna, finely chopped celery, red onion, and shredded carrot. Add mayonnaise, Dijon mustard, salt, and pepper to taste.

◇ Blend the ingredients thoroughly until the tuna salad is uniformly mixed.

◇ Top the tuna salad with optional items such as cucumber slices, avocado slices, cherry tomatoes, or fresh parsley.

◇ Fold the lettuce leaves to form wraps around the tuna salad and any extras you like to include.

Greek Quinoa Salad

Ingredients:
- One cup of washed and cooked quinoa, per package directions
- Half red onion, coarsely chopped
- Half cup chopped and pitted Kalamata olives
- One cup chopped cherry tomatoes
- Half a cup of crumbled feta cheese,
- One tablespoon of red wine vinegar,
- One teaspoon of dried oregano
- One cup of chopped fresh parsley
- One cup of extra virgin olive oil.
- Season with salt and pepper

- Garnish with lemon slices, if desired

Instructions:
◇ Wash quinoa in cold water and cook as directed on the package. Let it cool.

◇ Place cooked quinoa, diced cucumber, half cherry tomatoes, red onion, feta cheese, crumbled, sliced Kalamata olives, and chopped fresh parsley in a big bowl.

◇ To make the dressing, combine the extra-virgin olive oil, red wine vinegar, dried oregano, salt, and pepper in a small bowl.

◇ Pour the dressing over the combination of quinoa. Toss lightly to coat all items equally.

◇ Use your taste buds to gauge how much salt and pepper you like.

◇ To allow the flavors to merge, chill the Greek Quinoa Salad in the refrigerator for at least half an hour, if possible.

Chicken and Vegetable Stir-Fry
Ingredients:
- One pound of thinly sliced, boneless, skinless chicken breast
- Two tablespoons of soy sauce (you may substitute low-sodium soy sauce if you like)
- One tablespoon of oyster sauce

- One tablespoon each of cornstarch and sesame
oil;
- Two tablespoons of vegetable oil
- Two minced garlic cloves
- One tablespoon of grated ginger
- One bell pepper, cut thinly
– One cup florets of broccoli
- One chopped carrot
- One cup of snap peas with the ends removed
- One cup of sliced mushrooms
- Two chopped green onions
- Prepared cooked quinoa or brown rice for serving
- Sesame seeds
- Finely chopped parsley or cilantro

Instructions:
◇ Place the chicken slices, soy sauce, oyster
sauce, and cornstarch in a bowl. Stir thoroughly
and let marinate for fifteen minutes or more.

◇ Heat the vegetable and sesame oils in a big
skillet or wok over medium-high heat.

◇ Put the chicken in the hot pan after marinating.
Stir-fry the chicken until it's cooked through and has
a subtle brown hue. Take chicken out of the skillet
and set it aside.

◇ If necessary, add a little extra vegetable oil to the
same wok. Grated ginger and garlic should be
sautéed until aromatic. Add the snap peas,
mushrooms, bell pepper, broccoli, and julienned

carrot. Keep Stir-frying the veggies until they become crispy tender

◇ Add the cooked chicken back to the wok and toss to mix it in with the veggies.

◇ Stir everything together after adding the chopped green onions.

◇ If necessary, add more salt or soy sauce to the seasoning.
◇ Garnish with chopped parsley or cilantro and sesame seeds.

MOUTH WATERING SOUPS

Lentil Soup

Ingredients:
- One cup of rinsed dried green or brown lentils
- One diced onion
- Two diced peeled carrots
- Two chopped celery stalks
- Three minced garlic cloves
- One 14-oz can of diced, undrained tomatoes
- Six cups of low-sodium vegetable broth - - One teaspoon each of ground cumin and coriander
- One-half tsp smoked paprika
- One bay leaf
-Two tablespoons of olive oil
- Salt and pepper to taste.

- Chopped fresh parsley (for garnish)
- Slabs of lemon (for serving)

Instructions:
- Heat the olive oil in a big pot over medium heat.
- Add the minced garlic, diced onion, diced carrots, and diced celery.
- Sauté the veggies till they get tender.
- Include the rinsed lentils in the pot with the aromatics and stir to mi
- Add the veggie broth that is reduced in sodium. Simmer the mixture for a while.
- Mix in the bay leaf, smoked paprika, ground coriander, cumin, and diced tomatoes (with their liquid).
- Lower the pot's temperature to a simmer, cover it, and allow the lentils to cook for 25 to 30 minutes, or until they are soft.
- Add salt and pepper to taste when preparing the soup. As necessary, adjust the seasonings.
- Before serving, dispose of the bay leaf.
- Add freshly chopped parsley as a garnish.
 - Lemon wedges alongside for a burst of citrus flavor.

Vegetable Soup

Ingredients:
- One chopped onion
- Two minced garlic cloves
- Two peeled and sliced carrots
- Two chopped celery stalks

- One chopped bell pepper,(any color)
- One diced zucchini
- One cup of chopped green beans
- One cup of frozen or fresh corn kernels
- One 14-oz can of diced tomatoes
- Eight cups of low-sodium vegetable broth - One teaspoon of dried oregano and thyme
- To taste, add salt and pepper.
- Two teaspoons of olive oil.
- Chopped fresh parsley (for garnish)
- Optional grated Parmesan cheese for serving

Instructions:
- Heat the olive oil in a big pot over medium heat. Add minced garlic and chopped onion. The onion should be sautéed until transparent.
- Include diced bell pepper, diced zucchini, sliced carrots, sliced celery, green beans, and corn in the saucepan. Mix everything together.
- Add the veggie broth that is low in sodium. Simmer the mixture for a while.
- Stir in the dried oregano, dried thyme, and chopped tomatoes together with their liquid. Simmer until the vegetables are soft, 15 to 20 minutes.
- Add salt and pepper to taste when preparing the soup. As necessary, adjust the seasonings.
 - Add freshly chopped parsley as a garnish.
- You can add more taste by optionally sprinkling grated Parmesan cheese on top.

Fisherman's Stew

Ingredients:
- One pound of chunked white fish filets, such as halibut or cod
- One pound of peeled and deveined shrimp
- Diced onion
- Two minced garlic cloves
- One chopped bell pepper, any color
- One sliced celery stalk
- One chopped carrot
- Diced tomatoes
- Four cups of low-sodium vegetable or fish broth;
-Half a cup of dry white wine (optional)
- One teaspoon dried thyme
- Two tablespoons tomato paste
- One teaspoon paprika
-To taste, add salt and pepper.
- Two teaspoons of olive oil.
- Chopped fresh parsley (for garnish)
- Toasted bread (to be served)

Instructions:
- Warm up the olive oil in a pot over medium heat. Add the diced carrot, diced onion, diced celery, diced bell pepper, and minced garlic. Sauté the veggies till they get tender.
- Mix in the tomato paste and chopped tomatoes, along with their liquid. Simmer for a few minutes to bring out the flavors.
- Add white wine (if using) and low-sodium fish or veggie broth. Simmer the mixture for a while.

- Season the saucepan with salt, pepper, dried
thyme, and paprika. Mix everything together.
- Add the shrimp and fish chunks to the pot gently.
Simmer until the shrimp turn pink and the fish is
well done.
- Taste the stew and make any necessary
adjustments to the seasoning.
- Add freshly chopped parsley as a garnish.
- Crusty bread on the side (optional)

Chicken Noodle Soup

Ingredients:
- One pound of thinly sliced chicken breast
- Eight cups of low-sodium chicken broth
- Two minced garlic cloves
- One tablespoon of grated fresh ginger
- Two tablespoons of soy sauce
 (if preferred, use low-sodium soy sauce)
- One tablespoon each of sesame oil and rice
vinegar
- 4 ounces of rice noodles, or any other kind of
noodles
- One cup of sliced shiitake mushrooms
- One julienned carrot
- One cup of bean sprouts
- Two cups of chopped baby carrots
- Sliced green onions (for garnish)
- Chopped fresh cilantro (as a garnish)
- slices of lime (for serving)

Ingredients:
- Thinly slice the breast of chicken.
- Prepare the rice noodles as directed on the package. After draining, set away.
- Finely chop your garlic and finely grate your ginger in a big pot of sesame oil until aromatic.
- Place the sliced chicken in the saucepan and cook it until it loses its pink color.
- Add the rice vinegar, soy sauce, and low-sodium chicken broth. Simmer the mixture for a while.
- Include chopped baby carrot, and shiitake mushrooms in the pot. Simmer the veggies until they are soft.
-The cooked rice noodles should be added to the pot and stirred to mix.
- If necessary, add more salt or soy sauce to the seasoning.
- Add chopped cilantro, sliced green onions, and bean sprouts as garnish.

Broccoli Cheddar Soup

Ingredients:
One pound of freshly chopped broccoli, including the stems
- One chopped onion
- Two minced garlic cloves
- Four cups of low-sodium chicken or vegetable broth
- One medium-sized peeled and chopped potato
- Two cups of shredded sharp cheddar cheese
- Half a cup of whole or half-and-half milk

- Two tablespoons of butter
-Two tablespoons of all-purpose flour, salt, and pepper to taste.
- Add paprika or nutmeg for extra flavor
- Optional: bread or croutons to serve

Instructions:
- Melt butter in a pot over medium heat. Add minced garlic and chopped onion.
The onion should be sautéed until transparent.
- Add diced potato and chopped broccoli, including stems, to the pot. Mix well to include the aromatics.
- Add the low-sodium chicken or vegetarian broth and Simmer the mixture for a while.
- Lower the heat to a simmer, cover the pot, and let it sit there for the broccoli and potato to become cooked, around 15 to 20 minutes.
- Transfer the soup to a blender in batches or use an immersion blender. Blend till creamy and smooth.
- Melt the remaining butter in a different small pot over medium heat.
- Add all-purpose flour and stir to make a roux. Simmer for one to two minutes.
- Stirring continuously to prevent lumps, gradually add the roux to the blended soup.
- Add the shredded cheddar cheese and stir until it melts and is thoroughly mixed in.
- Add half-and-half or whole milk, stirring constantly.
- Add salt and pepper to taste when preparing the soup. If preferred, add a pinch of paprika or nutmeg for more taste.

- Let the soup warm through, and add extra milk or broth if necessary to change the consistency.

Carrot and Ginger Soup

Ingredients:
- One pound of peeled and sliced carrots
- One diced onion
- Two minced garlic cloves; one tablespoon of grated fresh ginger
- one tablespoon of olive oil
- Four cups of low-sodium vegetable broth - Diced and peeled medium potato
- One teaspoon of ground turmeric
- One can (about fourteen ounces) of coconut milk (optional, for creaminess)
- Salt and pepper to taste
- Fresh parsley or cilantro (to garnish)

Instructions:
- Warm up the olive oil in a big pot over medium heat. Put the grated ginger, minced garlic, and diced onion. The onion should be sautéed until transparent.
- Include diced potatoes and sliced carrots in the stew. Mix well to include the aromatics.
- Add the veggie broth that is low in sodium.
- Simmer the mixture
 - Lower the heat to a simmer, cover the saucepan, and allow the carrots and potato to cook for 20 to 25 minutes, or until they are soft.

- Transfer the soup to a blender in batches or use an immersion blender. Blend till creamy and smooth.
- Mix in the optional coconut milk for creaminess and the ground turmeric for color. Blend thoroughly.
- Add salt and pepper to taste when preparing the soup. As necessary, adjust the seasonings.
- If any more ingredients were added, let the soup warm all the way through.

Cauliflower Leek Soup

Ingredients:
- One big cauliflower, divided into pieces
- Two cleaned and thinly sliced leeks (only the white and light green portions)
- One chopped onion;
- Two minced garlic cloves
- Four cups of low-sodium vegetable broth
- Diced and peeled medium potato
- Two tablespoons olive oil
- One teaspoon fresh or dried thyme
- Season with salt and pepper to suit. You may also add chopped chives or Greek yogurt or cream as a garnish.

Instructions:
- Warm up the olive oil in a big pot over medium heat. Add the sliced leeks and diced onion. Sauté the food until it becomes tender.
- Add the minced thyme and garlic to the pot. Sauté for about 1 more minute.

- Include the chopped potato and cauliflower florets
in the saucepan.
Mix everything together.
- Add the veggie broth that is reduced in sodium.
Simmer the mixture for a while.
- Lower the heat to a simmer, cover the saucepan,
and leave the soup for 20 to 25 minutes, or until the
potato and cauliflower are soft.
- Transfer the soup to a blender in batches or use
an immersion blender. Blend till creamy and
smooth.
- Add salt and pepper to taste when preparing the
soup.
- provide chopped chives as a garnish to provide a
pop of freshness.

Spinach and Quinoa Soup

Ingredients:
- One cup of washed quinoa
- One chopped onion
- One tablespoon olive oil
- Two minced garlic cloves
- One chopped carrot
- One sliced celery stalk
- One teaspoon each of ground cumin and
coriander
- Chopped fresh spinach
- 6 cups low-sodium vegetable broth
- Lemon wedges (to serve)
- Salt & pepper to taste

Instructions:
- Place the quinoa in a bowl and run cold water over
- Warm up the olive oil in a big pot over medium heat. Add the celery, carrot, sliced onion, and minced garlic. Sauté the veggies till they get tender.
- After adding the ground coriander and cumin, give them a minute to roast.
- Fill the saucepan with the low-sodium vegetable broth after adding the rinsed quinoa. Simmer the mixture for a while.
- Lower the heat to a simmer, cover the pot, and leave it there for the quinoa to cook, which should take around 15 to 20 minutes.
- Add the freshly chopped spinach and heat through until it wilts.
- Add salt and pepper to taste when preparing the soup. As necessary, adjust the seasonings.
- Lemon wedges alongside.

Pumpkin Soup

Ingredients
- Two cups pumpkin puree (canned or homemade)
- One chopped onion
- Two minced garlic cloves
- One diced carrot
- One peeled and diced apple
- Four cups of low-sodium chicken or veggie broth
- One teaspoon of ground cinnamon
- One and a half teaspoons of ground ginger and nutmeg

- One tablespoon olive oil
- Season to taste with salt and pepper
- Greek yogurt or cream as a garnish
- Pumpkin seeds as an optional topping

Instructions:
- Place olive oil in a big saucepan and heat it to medium heat. Cook the chopped onion until it becomes tender.
- Include ground ginger, cinnamon, and nutmeg as well as chopped garlic. Sauté until aromatic, about 1 minute.
- Include diced apple and carrot in the saucepan. After a few minutes, stir and continue cooking until the vegetables begin to soften.
- Add the pureed pumpkin after adding the vegetable or chicken broth. Mix thoroughly to blend.
- Lower the soup's temperature to a simmer. After the vegetables are soft, cover and cook for 15 to 20 minutes.
- Transfer the soup to a blender in batches or use an immersion blender. Blend till creamy and smooth.
- Add salt and pepper to taste when preparing the soup. Taste and adjust the seasonings.
- Add pumpkin seeds as a crisp garnish (optional)

Chicken and Rice Soup

Ingredients:
- Shredded chicken breast
- One cup of chopped carrots

- One cup of diced celery
- One cup chopped onions
- Two minced garlic cloves
- One cup cooked white or brown rice
- One bay leaf
- Eight cups low-sodium chicken broth
- One teaspoon dried thyme
- Season with salt and pepper
- Finely slice fresh parsley (for garnish)

Instructions:
- Bake or boil the chicken breast until it is done. Cut the chicken into small shreds.
- Chop the onion, celery, and carrots
-Add the minced garlic and continue to sauté until the veggies are tender.
- Add the dried thyme and bay leaf to the low-sodium chicken broth. Simmer the mixture for a while.
- Fill the pot with the shredded chicken.
To allow the flavors to mingle, boil the soup for fifteen to twenty minutes.
- Stir thoroughly after adding the cooked rice to the broth. After 10 more minutes of simmering, the rice should be well heated.
- Add salt and pepper to taste when preparing the soup. As necessary, adjust the seasonings.
- Before serving, dispose of the bay leaf.
 - For extra freshness, garnish with freshly chopped parsley.

Quinoa and Kale Soup

Ingredients:
- One cup rinsed quinoa
- One bunch chopped kale with stems removed
- One diced onion
- Two peeled and diced carrots
- Two diced celery stalks
- Three minced garlic cloves
- One 14-oz can of diced, undrained tomatoes
- Two tablespoons of olive oil
- 1 teaspoon each of ground cumin and dried thyme
- One bay leaf
- Eight cups of low-sodium vegetable broth
-Add Salt and pepper to taste
-Lemon juice (Serve fresh)
- Chopped fresh parsley (for garnish)

Instructions:
- Warm up the olive oil in a pot over medium heat. Add the minced garlic, diced onion, diced carrots, and diced celery. Sauté the veggies till they get tender.
- Include the rinsed quinoa in the pot and mix it in with the veggies by stirring.
- Add the veggie broth that is low in sodium. Add the bay leaf, ground cumin, and dry thyme. Simmer the mixture for a while.
- Lower the heat to a simmer, cover the saucepan, and leave it there for the quinoa to cook, which should take around 15 to 20 minutes.

- Mix in diced tomatoes along with their liquid. Cook the kale until it begins to wilt.
- Add salt and pepper to taste when preparing the soup. As necessary, adjust the seasonings.
- Remove the bay leaf prior to serving.
- Add freshly chopped parsley as a garnish.
– Pour freshly squeezed lemon juice into each bowl to add a zesty taste.

Mushroom Barley Soup

Ingredients:
- One cup of washed pearl barley
- Eight cups low-sodium vegetable or mushroom broth
- One diced onion
- Two diced peeled carrots
- Eight ounces of sliced button or cremini mushrooms
- Two diced celery stalks
- Three minced garlic cloves
- A teaspoon of thyme, dried
- One bay leaf, two tablespoons of olive oil, and salt & pepper to taste
- Chopped fresh parsley (for garnish)

Instructions:
- Heat the olive oil in a pot over medium heat. Add the minced garlic, diced onion, diced carrots, and diced celery. Sauté the veggies till they get tender.

- Add the sliced mushrooms to the pot and sauté them until they begin to brown and release their moisture.
- Use cold water to rinse the pearl barley. Stir it into the pot after adding the vegetables.
- Add the mushroom or vegetable broth. Add the bay leaf and the dried thyme. Simmer the mixture for a while.
- Lower the pot's temperature to a simmer, cover it, and wait for the barley to become tender, around 40 to 45 minutes.
- Add salt and pepper to taste when preparing the soup.
- Add freshly cut parsley as a garnish.

Butternut Squash Soup

Ingredients:
-A medium-sized butternut squash that has been peeled, seeded, and diced
- One diced onion
- Two carrots that have been peeled and chopped
- Two apples that have been peeled, cored, and chopped
- Three minced garlic cloves
- Four cups vegetable broth with minimal sodium
- One teaspoon ground cinnamon
- One-half tsp freshly ground nutmeg
- One-fourth tsp ground ginger
- One cup of unsweetened almond milk (or your favorite milk)
- Two tablespoons of olive oil

- Salt & pepper to taste
- Fresh leaves of thyme (for garnish)
- Pepitas, or pumpkin seeds (for garnish)

Instructions:
- Cut the butternut squash into dice and remove the seeds. Dice the onion; peel, core, and chop the carrots; chop the apples.
- Warm up the olive oil in a big pot over medium heat. Add minced garlic and chopped onion. The onion should be sautéed until transparent.
- Include chopped apples, carrots, and diced butternut squash in the saucepan. Mix well to include the aromatics.
- Add the veggie broth that is reduced in sodium. Simmer the mixture for a while.
- Fill the saucepan with ground ginger, ground nutmeg, ground cinnamon, and salt and pepper. Mix thoroughly to blend.
- After lowering the heat to low and covering the saucepan, simmer the vegetables for 20 to 25 minutes, or until they are soft.
- Blend the soup with an immersion blender or divide it into batches in a blender. Process till smooth.
- To get the right consistency, stir with unsweetened almond milk or any other chosen milk.
- After tasting the soup, modify the seasoning.

Tomato Basil Soup

Ingredients:
- One 28-ounce can of whole peeled tomatoes without water
- One chopped onion
- Three minced garlic cloves
- Half cup finely chopped fresh basil leaves - Two cups low-sodium vegetable broth
- One-fourth cup olive oil
- One teaspoon of oregano, dried
- One teaspoon of sugar, if desired to counteract the acidity.
- Half cup heavy cream (optional for a creamier version)
- Salt & pepper to taste
- Parmesan cheese, grated (as a garnish)
- Fresh sprigs of basil (to garnish)

Instructions:
- Heat the olive oil in a pot over medium heat. Add minced garlic and chopped onion. The onion should be sautéed until transparent.
- Fill the saucepan with the whole peeled tomatoes along with their juice. Using a spoon, tear apart the tomatoes.
- Add the dried oregano and low-sodium vegetable broth. Simmer the mixture for a while.
- Blend the soup in batches in a blender or with an immersion blender. Process till smooth.
-Add chopped fresh basil leaves and stir. Simmer further for about ten to fifteen minutes.

- Add salt and pepper to taste when preparing the soup. You can optionally add sugar to counteract the tomatoes' acidity.
- To achieve a creamier texture, whisk in the heavy cream if preferred.
- Let the soup warm through, giving it a little stir now and then.
- Add grated Parmesan cheese as a garnish.

CHAPTER FOUR

TEAS

1. Nettle Leaf Tea

This tea has a high mineral and vitamin content. It might promote general wellbeing and health.

2. Ginger and Lemon Tea:

Make a warming and energizing tea by combining fresh ginger and lemon. The *3 anti-inflammatory* qualities of ginger are enhanced by the pleasant taste of lemon.

3. Rosehip Hibiscus Tea:

This antioxidant-rich tea contains hibiscus and rosehips, which may give you a quick vitamin C boost. It tastes tangy and fruity.

4. Peppermint Tea:

Well-known for its digestive advantages, peppermint tea is a delightful, caffeine-free beverage.

5. **Turmeric with Green Tea:**

For its anti-inflammatory qualities, mix a little bit of turmeric into a cup of green tea. Curcumin, which is present in turmeric, may be beneficial to health.

DESSERTS

Roasted Almond Stuffed Dates

Ingredients:
- Pitted Medjool dates
- Whole almonds, roasted or raw
- Optional: Coconut shreds for coating

Instructions
- Preheat the oven to 350°F (180°C) if using raw almonds.
- Gently cut each date in half lengthwise and extract the pit.
- Make sure each date's cavity is firmly packed with a whole almond.
- Arrange raw almonds on a baking sheet and roast for 8 to 10 minutes, or until they begin to turn a light golden color. Give them time to cool.
- To add even more flavor, coat the packed dates in shredded coconut, if preferred.

Baked Cinnamon Banana Chips

Ingredients:
- Mature bananas
- Lemon juice (recommended)
- Cinnamon powder
- (Optional) For sweetness, add honey or maple syrup.

Instructions:
- Set the oven temperature to 200°F, or 93°C.
- Peel and thinly slice the bananas into rounds. If you want to keep the banana slices from browning, you can delicately spray them with lemon juice.
- Arrange the banana slices in a single layer, making sure they are not in contact with one another, on a baking sheet covered with parchment paper.
- Drizzle the banana slices with ground cinnamon. Adjust the quantity to your taste.
- You can drizzle a little honey or maple syrup over the banana slices if you'd like them to be even sweeter.
After the banana slices
- Bake the banana chips for two to three hours, or until they are crisp, in a preheated oven. Watch them closely, and turn the baking sheet over if needed.

Grilled Pineapple Slices

Ingredients:
- Raw pineapple - Optional honey or maple syrup for sprinkling
- Optional cinnamon (for dusting)

Instructions:
- Turn the heat up to medium-high on your grill.
- Cut the pineapple into rings or spears after peeling it.

- Directly place the pineapple slices onto the grill grates that have been preheated. Cook the pineapple for two to three minutes on each side, or until grill marks appear and it begins to gently caramelize.
- Drizzle the grilled pineapple slices with honey or maple syrup if you'd like a little sweetness.(Optional)
- Sprinkle cinnamon on top of the grilled pineapple pieces for an additional flavorful explosion.
- Take the pineapple off the grill once the outside has some caramelization and grill marks.

Avocado Chocolate Mousse

Ingredients:
- A pair of mature avocados
- One-fourth cup powdered cocoa
- One-fourth cup honey or maple syrup
- One tsp vanilla extract
- A pinch of salt
- An optional garnish of chopped almonds, fresh berries, or cocoa powder

Instructions:
- Scoop the flesh into a food processor or blender after cutting the ripe avocados in half and removing the pits.
- Fill the food processor or blender with chocolate powder.
- Add honey or maple syrup for sweetness.

- To bring out the flavors, add a dash of salt and vanilla extract.
- Process all the ingredients in a blender until a creamy, smooth consistency is reached. If necessary, scrape down the sides.
- Refrigerate the ingredients for approximately 30 minutes to achieve a cooler mousse.
- Add fresh berries, sliced almonds, or a sprinkle of cocoa powder

Fruit Salad with Mint

Ingredients:
- One cup of fresh blueberries
- Two cups of freshly hulled and sliced strawberries
- One cup chopped fresh pineapple
- One cup diced fresh mango
- One cup of chopped green grapes
- One tablespoon of finely chopped fresh mint leaves
- One tablespoon of honey (optional, for a hint of sweetness)

Instructions:
- As needed, wash and prepare each fruit. Cut grapes in half, dice mango and pineapple, then slice strawberries.
- Place the sliced strawberries, blueberries, chopped pineapple, diced mango, and halved grapes in a large mixing dish.
- Top the fruit mixture with the finely chopped fresh mint leaves.

- Drizzle honey over the fruit salad and toss lightly to mix, if you'd like a little sweetness.
- Gently toss the fruit salad to distribute the optional sugar and mint evenly.
- Before serving, chill a chilled fruit salad in the refrigerator for approximately half an hour.

Baked Apples with Cinnamon

Ingredients:
- Four medium-sized apples, such Honeycrisp or Granny Smith
- Two teaspoons of melted unsalted butter
- Two tablespoons maple syrup or brown sugar
- One teaspoon of ground cinnamon
- One-fourth cup of chopped nuts (for garnish, if desired)
- Greek yogurt or vanilla ice cream (optional; used to serve)

Instructions:
- Adjust the oven temperature to 375°F (190°C).
- Clean and core the apples. To make a well for the filling, you can leave the bottom in place.
- Combine melted butter, ground cinnamon, and brown sugar or maple syrup in a small bowl.
- The cored apples should be put in a baking dish. Fill the center of each apple with a spoonful of the cinnamon mixture.
- You can choose to top the cinnamon mixture with chopped nuts, like pecans or walnuts.

- Bake the apples for around 25 to 30 minutes, or until they are soft, in a preheated oven. Depending on the size and kind of apples, the baking time can change.
- Apples topped with Greek yogurt or a scoop of vanilla ice cream.

Greek Yogurt with Honey and Walnuts

Ingredients:
- One cup of Greek yogurt
- Two teaspoons of honey
- Two tablespoons of walnuts, chopped

Instructions:
- Split the Greek yogurt, honey, and walnuts into equal portions.
- Transfer the Greek yogurt into a serving dish using a spoon.
- Drizzle the Greek yogurt with honey. Depending on how sweet you want your food, adjust the amount.
- Top the yogurt and honey with a small handful of chopped walnuts.
- To ensure an equitable distribution, you can optionally use a spoon to gently swirl the honey and walnuts into the Greek yogurt.

Watermelon Sorbet

Ingredients:

- Four cups cubed, seedless watermelon
- One-fourth cup honey or maple syrup (modify according to desired level of sweetness)
- One tsp squeezed lemon or lime juice
- Mint leaves as an optional garnish

Instructions:
- After removing all seeds, cut the seedless watermelon into tiny pieces.
- Arrange the watermelon cubes in a single layer on a baking sheet that has been lined with parchment paper. Freeze the watermelon for a minimum of three to four hours, or until it is fully frozen.
- Place the frozen watermelon cubes, honey (or maple syrup), and lemon or lime juice in a food processor or blender.
- Blend the concoction into a creamy, smooth consistency. It might be necessary to pause and scrape down the sides several times.
- If necessary, add additional honey or maple syrup after tasting the sorbet to make it sweeter.

Poached Pears with Vanilla Yogurt

Ingredients:
- Two cups water
- One cup red wine (or grape juice for a non-alcoholic version)
- Four ripe pears, peeled and cut in half
- Half a cup of maple syrup or honey
- One vanilla bean or one teaspoon of vanilla extract

- One cinnamon stick
- Vanilla or Greek yogurt to be served
- Optional garnish: chopped mint leaves or almonds

Instructions:
- Peel and cut the pears in half, taking off the core.
- Put water, red wine (or grape juice), maple syrup or honey, cinnamon stick, and vanilla bean seeds (or vanilla extract) in a pot.
- Put the pear halves into the liquid used for poaching. The pears should be poached for 15 to 20 minutes, or until they are soft but not mushy, by gently simmering them.
- Take the pears out of the liquid used for poaching and let them cool a little.
- Simmer the poaching liquid until it thickens and reduces to a syrup consistency, if preferred.
- Present the Poached Pears beside a generous portion of vanilla or Greek yogurt.
- For an added touch, garnish with chopped nuts or mint leaves.

A Mixed Berry Parfait

Ingredients:
- One cup of mixed berries, including blackberries, raspberries, blueberries, and strawberries
- One cup of Greek yogurt
- Two teaspoons of maple syrup or honey
- Granola for stacking
- Optional fresh mint leaf garnish

Instructions:
- Clean and get ready the mixed berries. Slice and hull the strawberries, if using.
- Combine the Greek yogurt and maple syrup in a bowl. To taste, adjust the sweetness.
- Begin by layering Greek yogurt into serving bowls or glasses.
- Cover the yogurt with a layer of mixed berries.
- Continue layering until the top of the glass is reached, and then add a layer of berries to complete.
- To add more crunch and texture, sprinkle granola over the top layer.

Cocoa-Dusted Almonds

Ingredients:
- One cup whole almonds
- One tablespoon chocolate powder without sugar added
- One-fourth teaspoon vanilla extract
- Two tablespoons powdered sugar
- A dash of salt

Instructions:
- Toast the almonds for five to seven minutes, tossing often, over medium heat in a dry skillet, until aromatic. Take care not to scorch them.
- Combine the powdered sugar, vanilla extract, cocoa powder, and a little pinch of salt in a bowl.
- Toss the almonds in the cocoa mixture until they are evenly coated, while they are still warm.

- Let the almonds that have been sprinkled with
cocoa cool fully.

Pumpkin Oat Cookies

Ingredients:
- One cup of canned pumpkin puree
- Half a cup of softened unsalted butter
- Half a cup of packed brown sugar
- One-fourth cup of sugar, granulated
- One big egg
- One tsp vanilla extract
- Half cups of steel-cut oats
- One cup flour (all-purpose)
- Half a teaspoon of baking soda
- Half a teaspoon of ground cinnamon
- One-fourth teaspoon of nutmeg, ground
- One-fourth teaspoon of salt
- Half cup chocolate chips or raisins,
if desired

Instructions:
- Turn the oven's temperature up to 350°F (175°C).
Use parchment paper to line baking sheets.
- Cream the softened butter, brown sugar, and
granulated sugar in a big bowl until they are light
and fluffy.
- Stir the egg into the creamed mixture along with
the canned pumpkin puree. Blend thoroughly.
- Mix the oats, flour, baking soda, nutmeg,
cinnamon, and salt in a separate basin. Add these

dry ingredients to the wet mixture gradually and stir until thoroughly blended.
- If preferred, mix chocolate chips or raisins into the cookie batter.
- Place rounded scoops of cookie dough, allowing space between each, onto the baking sheets that have been prepared.
- Bake for 12 to 15 minutes, or until the sides are golden brown, in a preheated oven.

Baked Peaches with Almond Crumble

Ingredients:
- Four ripe peaches, pitted and halved
- Two tablespoons maple syrup or honey
- One tsp of vanilla extract

Almond Crumble:
- Half cup almond flour
- One-fourth cup rolled oats
- Two tablespoons brown sugar or coconut sugar
- Two tablespoons unsalted butter or melted coconut oil
- One-half teaspoon ground cinnamon
- A dash of salt

Instructions:
- Turn the oven's temperature up to 375°F (190°C).
- Cut the ripe ones in half and remove the pits. Transfer them to a baking dish, cut side up.
- Sprinkle vanilla extract and honey (or maple syrup) over the peaches.

- Almond flour, rolled oats, brown sugar or coconut sugar, melted butter or coconut oil, crushed cinnamon, and a pinch of salt. Stir until a crumbly consistency is achieved.
- An even spoon over the peach halves the mixture of almond crumble.
- Bake for 20 to 25 minutes, or until the crumble is golden brown and the peaches are soft, in a preheated oven.
- Before serving, let the baked peaches with almond crumble cool somewhat.

Coconut Date Balls

Ingredients:
- Four ripe peaches, pitted and halved
- Two tablespoons maple syrup or honey
- One tsp of vanilla extract

- Half cup almond flour
- One-fourth cup rolled oats
- Two tablespoons brown sugar or coconut sugar
- Two tablespoons unsalted butter or melted coconut oil
- Half teaspoon ground cinnamon
- A dash of salt

Instructions:
- Turn the oven's temperature up to 375°F (190°C).
- Cut the ripe ones in half and remove the pits. Transfer them to a baking dish, cut side up.

- Sprinkle vanilla extract and honey (or maple syrup) over the peaches.
- Almond flour, rolled oats, brown sugar or coconut sugar, melted butter or coconut oil, crushed cinnamon, and a pinch of salt. Stir until a crumbly consistency is achieved.
- An even spoon over the peach halves the mixture of almond crumble.
- Bake for 20 to 25 minutes, or until the crumble is golden brown and the peaches are soft, in a preheated - Before serving, let the baked peaches with almond crumble cool somewhat.

Banana Ice Cream

Ingredients
- Four ripe bananas, cut, frozen, and peeling
- One teaspoon of optional vanilla extract

Instructions:
- Ripe bananas. After lining a tray or plate with parchment paper, place the banana slices on it and freeze for at least two to three hours, or overnight.
- After the banana slices are frozen, put them in a food processor or blender. If desired, add vanilla extract.
- Purée the frozen bananas according to your preference. It might be necessary to stop and scrape down the food processor or blender sides several times.
- For a soft-serve consistency, serve the banana ice cream right away. To get a more solid consistency,

move the ice cream into a container and place it in
the freezer for 1-2 hours
- Add your preferred garnishes, like honey,
shredded coconut, or chopped nuts.

NUTRITIOUS DINNER

Grilled Shrimp Tacos with Cabbage Slaw

Ingredients:
- Two tablespoons olive oil
- One teaspoon chili powder
- One pound of large shrimp, peeled and deveined
- Half a teaspoon each of cumin and paprika
- One lime's juice;
- Salt and pepper to taste

Cabbage Slaw:
- Two cups of purple or green shredded cabbage
- 1/4 cup chopped cilantro
- One julienned carrot
- 1/4 cup of Greek yogurt, plain
- One tablespoon of mayo
- One lime's juice
- To taste, add salt and pepper.

Tacos:
- Tiny tortillas made from corn or whole wheat
- Optional toppings include chopped tomatoes, salsa, and sliced avocado.

Instructions:
- Shrimp, lime juice, chili powder, cumin, paprika, and olive oil should all be combined in a bowl.

Once well coated, toss and let marinate for 15 to 20 minutes.
- Turn the heat to medium-high on a grill or grill pan.
- Put marinated shrimp straight onto the grill or skewer them. Shrimp should be cooked through and opaque after two to three minutes on each side of the grill.
- Shredded cabbage, diced carrot, chopped cilantro, Greek yogurt, mayonnaise, lime juice, salt, and pepper should all be combined in a different bowl. Toss until thoroughly mixed.
- Spoon cooked shrimp into each tortilla, then cover with cabbage slaw.
- You can add extras like chopped tomatoes, salsa, or sliced avocado.

Spinach and Feta Stuffed Turkey Burgers

Ingredients:
- One pound of lean ground turkey
- One cup of chopped fresh spinach
 half a cup of crumbled feta cheese
- One-fourth cup of finely chopped red onion
- Two minced cloves of garlic
- One teaspoon of oregano, dried
- To taste, add salt and pepper
- Use olive oil while grilling

Regarding toppings:
- Burger buns made of whole wheat

- Sliced tomatoes
- Rings of red onion
- Fresh spinach leaves
- Greek yogurt or tzatziki sauce for serving

Instructions:
- Turn the heat up to medium-high on an outdoor grill or grill pan.
- Ground turkey, chopped spinach, crumbled feta, minced garlic, red onion, dried oregano, salt, and pepper should all be combined in a big bowl. Blend until thoroughly blended.
- Create equal quantities of the ingredients and shape them into burger patties.
- Make a well in the middle of each patty and add a tiny bit of feta. Reshape the burger and enclose the cheese.
- To keep the patties from sticking, lightly coat the grill grates with olive oil. The turkey patties should be cooked through and have an internal temperature of 165°F (74°C) after grilling them for about 5 to 7 minutes on each side.
- You can grill the whole wheat burger buns for the final few minutes.
- Top the toasted buns with the grilled turkey patties. Add sliced tomatoes, red onion rings, a dollop of Greek yogurt or tzatziki sauce, and fresh spinach leaves on top.

Whole Grain Pasta with Tomato and Spinach Sauce

Ingredients:
- Two tablespoons olive oil
- Three chopped cloves of garlic
- Eight ounces whole grain pasta
- One can (14 oz) fire-roasted chopped tomatoes (for flavor)
- Two cups of fresh spinach leaves, cut and cleaned
- Half teaspoon each of dried oregano and basil
- Salt and pepper to taste
- Grated Parmesan cheese for decoration (optional)
- Optional fresh basil leaves as a garnish

Instructions:
- Cook the whole grain pasta until al dente, following the directions on the package. After draining, set away.
- Heat olive oil in a big skillet over medium heat. Once aromatic, add the minced garlic and sauté it for one to two minutes.
- Add the diced tomatoes to the skillet along with their liquid. Add the salt, pepper, dried basil, and oregano. Mix everything together.
- Simmer the sauce for ten to fifteen minutes, so that the flavors can combine and the sauce becomes a little thicker.
- Stir the freshly chopped spinach into the sauce until it wilts.

- Add the cooked whole grain pasta, spinach sauce, and tomato to the skillet. Toss until all of the sauce is well spread over the spaghetti.

Baked Chicken Breast with Sweet Potato and Broccoli

Ingredients:
- Four skinless and boneless chicken breasts
- One teaspoon of garlic powder
- Two tablespoons of olive oil
- One teaspoon powdered onion
- A teaspoon of thyme, dried
- To taste, add salt and pepper.

For broccoli and sweet potatoes:
- Two cups broccoli florets
- Two tablespoons olive oil
- Two medium-sized sweet potatoes, peeled and diced
- Adjust with salt and pepper to taste.
You may also add 1 teaspoon of paprika for flavor.

Instructions:
- Set the oven temperature to 400°F, or 200°C.
- Arrange the breasts of chicken on a baking sheet. Add a drizzle of olive oil and season with salt, pepper, dried thyme, onion powder, and garlic powder. Take care to coat the chicken breasts evenly.

- Combine the chopped sweet potatoes and broccoli florets with olive oil in another bowl. Add optional seasonings (salt, pepper, and paprika
- Place the broccoli and sweet potatoes on one side of the baking sheet and the seasoned chicken breasts on the other.
- Bake in the preheated oven for 25 to 30 minutes, or until the veggies are soft and the chicken is cooked through, reaching an internal temperature of 165°F or 74°C.
- Make sure the chicken juices run clear and the sweet potatoes are fork-tender.

Salmon and Quinoa Patties

Ingredients:
- One-fourth cup whole wheat bread crumbs
- One cup cooked quinoa
- One can (14 oz) pink salmon, drained and flakes
- One large egg
- One teaspoon Dijon mustard
- Two tablespoons finely chopped fresh parsley;
- One cup finely chopped red onion
- One lemon zest
- To taste, add salt and pepper
- Use olive oil while cooking

Instructions:
- Place cooked quinoa and drained, flaked salmon into a big bowl.

- Fill the bowl with breadcrumbs, lime zest, Dijon mustard, sliced red onion, red bell pepper, fresh parsley, and salt and pepper. Blend thoroughly.
- Break open the egg and whisk the mixture until everything is thoroughly mixed. To bind the patties together, use the egg.
- Create equal parts of the ingredients and form them into patties.
- In a skillet set over medium heat, warm up the olive oil.
- Add the salmon and quinoa patties to the skillet and cook, turning occasionally, for 3 to 4 minutes on each side, or until cooked through and golden brown.

Baked Cod with Lemon and Herbs

Ingredients:
- Four 6 ounce cod filets
- Two tablespoons each of fresh lemon juice and olive oil
- One lemon's zest
- Two minced garlic cloves
- One teaspoon of oregano, dried
- A teaspoon of thyme, dried
- Add salt and pepper to taste
- fresh parsley for garnishing desired

Instructions:
- Set the oven's temperature to 400°F, or 200°C.
- After using a paper towel to pat dry, put the cod filets in a baking dish.

- Olive oil, fresh lemon juice, zest, minced garlic, dried oregano, dried thyme, salt, and pepper should all be combined in a small bowl.
- Make sure the fish filets are thoroughly coated by pouring the lemon-herb marinade over them. Give them a good fifteen to twenty minutes to marinade.
- Bake the cod for around 12 to 15 minutes, or until a fork can easily pierce the fish.
- Make sure the cod is cooked all the way through and opaque.
- You can add some fresh parsley as a garnish if you'd like.

Baked Sweet Potato and Black Bean Enchiladas

Ingredients:
- One can (15 oz) of rinsed and drained black beans
- Two medium-sized sweet potatoes, peeled and chopped
- One cup of fresh corn kernels (frozen)
- One cup of chopped bell peppers, any hue
- One teaspoon of chili powder and cumin each
- To taste, salt and pepper
- Roasting olive oil

For the Sauce Enchilada:
- One 15-oz can of tomato sauce
- One teaspoon of chili powder and cumin each
- One-half teaspoon powdered garlic
To taste, add salt and pepper.

- Eight corn or whole wheat tortillas
- One cup of shredded cheese (you can use
Mexican mix or cheddar).
- Optional fresh cilantro garnish
- Sour cream or Greek yogurt for serving (optional)

Instructions:
- Turn the oven's temperature up to 375°F (190°C).
- Add diced sweet potatoes, olive oil, chili powder,
cumin, and salt & pepper to taste. Bake for 20 to 25
minutes, Baked through.
- Add the tomato sauce, cumin, garlic powder, chili
powder, and salt and pepper to a saucepan. Warm
the sauce thoroughly over medium heat.
- Roasted sweet potatoes, black beans, corn, sliced
bell peppers, cumin, chili powder, salt, and pepper
should all be combined in a big bowl. Blend
thoroughly.
- To make the tortillas more malleable, gently warm
them up. Fill each tortilla with a spoonful of filling,
roll each one up, and put seam-side down in a
baking tray.
- Drizzle the enchilada sauce that has been made
over the tortillas that have been rolled.
- Drizzle the enchiladas with shredded cheese.
- Bake for 20 to 25 minutes, or until the cheese is
bubbling and melted, in a preheated oven.
- You can add fresh cilantro as a garnish if you'd
like. Serve the Black Bean and Sweet Potato
Enchiladas hot out of the oven.

Vegetarian Chili with Kidney Beans

Ingredients:
- Two tsp olive oil
- One large onion, chopped
- Three minced garlic cloves
- One chopped bell pepper, any color
- One chopped zucchini
- One diced carrot
- Finely chopped and seeded jalapeño (optional for added heat)
- Two cans (15 oz each) of washed and drained kidney beans
- One can (28 ounces) of crushed tomatoes - One can (14 ounces) of diced tomatoes with fire-roasted taste
- One cup of fresh corn kernels or frozen
- One tablespoon chili powder
- Two tablespoons tomato paste
- Two teaspoons powdered cumin
- One tsp of paprika with smoke
- One teaspoon of oregano, dried
- Two cups of vegetable broth
- Toppings of fresh cilantro (optional)
- Salt and pepper to taste
- Optional grated cheese for topping
- Sour cream or Greek yogurt for serving (optional)

Instructions:
- Warm up the olive oil in a big pot over medium heat. Add the bell pepper, zucchini, carrot, onion,

and jalapeño chopped. Simmer the vegetables for 5
to 7 minutes, or until they are tender.
- Add salt, pepper, dried oregano, smoked paprika,
chili powder, and powdered cumin. Add the spices
and cook for a further two minutes to toast them.
- Fill the saucepan with kidney beans, chopped
tomatoes, crushed tomatoes, and tomato paste.
Toss to blend well.
- Add the veggie broth and boil the blend. For
twenty to twenty-five minutes, simmer over low heat
to enable flavors to mingle.
- Taste the chili and make any necessary
adjustments to the spices.

Mediterranean Chickpea Salad with Feta

Ingredients:
- Two cans of washed and drained chickpeas (15
ounces each).
- One diced cucumber
- One cup of chopped cherry tomatoes
- One finely chopped red onion
- One diced bell pepper of any color
- Half a cup of sliced Kalamata olives
- Half cup of feta cheese, crumbled
- Chopped fresh parsley as a garnish

Dressing:
- One teaspoon dried oregano
- Two teaspoons red wine vinegar
- One quarter cup extra virgin olive oil

- Add salt and pepper to taste
- Zest a lemon for extra crunch (optional)

Instructions:
- Give the tinned chickpeas a good rinse and drain.
Transfer them to a sizable mixing basin.
- Cut bell pepper, cucumber, cherry tomatoes in
half, finely chop red onion, and slice Kalamata
olives. Combine them with the chickpeas in the
bowl.
- Sprinkle the salad's components with crumbled
feta cheese.
- Combine the extra virgin olive oil, red wine
vinegar, dried oregano, salt, and pepper in a small
bowl. Zest the lemon if you want an extra zesty
burst.
- Over the salad components, drizzle the dressing.
Mix everything together gently until thoroughly
mixed.
- To allow the flavors to mingle, place the
Mediterranean Chickpea Salad in the refrigerator
for at least half an hour.

Roasted Turkey Breast with Brussels Sprouts

Ingredients:
- One 3- to 4-pound turkey breast with the skin and
bones intact
- Two tablespoons olive oil
- One teaspoon each of dried rosemary and thyme
- One teaspoon powdered garlic

To taste, add salt and pepper.

 Brussels Sprouts:
- One pound of chopped and halved
- Two teaspoons of olive oil
- Salt and pepper to taste

Instructions:
- Turn the oven's temperature up to 375°F (190°C).
- Use paper towels to pat the turkey breast dry.
Combine the olive oil, garlic powder, salt, pepper,
dried thyme, and dried rosemary in a small bowl.
- Evenly coat the turkey breast by rubbing it with
the olive oil and herb mixture.
- Combine salt, pepper, and olive oil with the halved
Brussels sprouts.
- Arrange the prepped Brussels sprouts around the
turkey breast, which should be placed in a roasting
pan or baking sheet.
- Roast the turkey for one to one and a half hours,
or until its internal temperature reaches 165°F
(74°C), in a preheated oven. When the Brussels
sprouts are soft and golden brown, they are done.
- Verify that the turkey's skin is brown and crispy
and that its fluids are clear.
- Before slicing, let the turkey rest for roughly ten
minutes. Juice retention is aided by this.

Eggplant Parmesan with Whole Wheat Pasta

Ingredients:
- One big eggplant, cut into rounds that are 1/2 inch thick.
- Salt to help eggplant sweat
- One cup all-purpose breadcrumbs
- Two beaten eggs
- Half cup grated Parmesan cheese
- Two cups marinara sauce (store-bought or homemade)
– Half cups shredded mozzarella cheese
- Optional fresh parsley or basil garnish

Whole Wheat Pasta:
- 8 oz. whole wheat pasta (you can use spaghetti or another type).
- Add salt to the water for pasta.
- Tossing with olive oil

Instructions:
- After putting the eggplant slices on a paper towel and seasoning them with salt, let them sweat for approximately half an hour. This aids in removing too much moisture.
- Turn the oven's temperature up to 375°F (190°C).
- Grated Parmesan and whole wheat breadcrumbs should be combined in a single bowl. Coat each eggplant slice with the breadcrumb mixture after dipping it in beaten eggs. After coating the slices,

put them on a baking sheet and bake for 20 to 25 minutes, or until they are crisp and golden.
- Cook the whole wheat pasta in salted water, following the directions on the package. To avoid sticking, drain and toss with a little olive oil.
- Apply a thin layer of marinara sauce to a baking dish. Place half of the slices of roasted eggplant on top of the sauce. Add extra marinara sauce on top, then half of the shredded mozzarella on top. With the remaining ingredients, repeat the stacking process.
- Bake for 25 to 30 minutes, or until the cheese is bubbling and melted, in a preheated oven.
- Make sure the cheese is browned and the eggplant is soft.
- If preferred, garnish with fresh parsley or basil.
- Spoon the whole wheat pasta over the eggplant parmesan.

Lemon Herb Grilled Chicken Breast

Ingredients:
- Four skinless and boneless chicken breasts
- One lemon's zest
- Two lemons juiced
- Two minced garlic cloves
- Three tablespoons of olive oil
- One teaspoon of dried rosemary
- One teaspoon of dried thyme
- One teaspoon of oregano, dried
- Add salt and pepper
- Optional fresh parsley for garnishing

Instructions:
- Lemon zest, lemon juice, olive oil, minced garlic, dried thyme, dried rosemary, dried oregano, salt, and pepper should all be combined in a bowl.
- Put the chicken breasts in a shallow dish or a plastic bag that can be sealed. Make sure every breast of chicken has a good coating by pouring the marinade over it. Let it marinate in the fridge for a minimum of half an hour, or for maximum flavor, two to four hours.
- Turn the heat up to medium-high.
- Take the chicken out of the marinade and let any extra to fall off. The internal temperature of the chicken breasts should reach 165°F (74°C) and the juices should run clear after grilling for approximately 6 to 8 minutes on each side.
- Make sure the chicken is thoroughly done, with no pink remaining in the middle.
- Prior to slicing, let the grilled chicken breasts have a few minutes of rest.
- If desired, garnish with fresh parsley.

Grilled Tofu and Vegetable Kebabs

Ingredients:
 Tofu Marinade:
- Two teaspoons soy sauce
- One tablespoon olive oil
- One tablespoon maple syrup or agave nectar;
- One teaspoon each of chopped garlic and ginger
- One teaspoon each of sesame oil and rice vinegar

- Salt and pepper to taste

Vegetable Kebabs:
- Cherry tomatoes
- Cut bell peppers into bits, any color
- Round slices of zucchini
- Diced red onion into wedges
- Cleaned and halved mushrooms
- Metal or wood skewers

Instructions:
- After pressing the tofu to squeeze out extra water, chop it into cubes.
- Combine soy sauce, sesame oil, rice vinegar, olive oil, maple syrup, chopped garlic, minced ginger, salt, and pepper in a bowl.
- Tofu cubes should be added to the marinade and let to marinate for at least 30 minutes
- Chop the vegetables into kebab-sized pieces and set aside while the tofu marinades.
- To add variation, alternately thread marinated tofu pieces and cooked veggies on skewers.
- Turn the heat up to medium-high on your grill.
- Grill the vegetable and tofu kebabs for ten to fifteen minutes, rotating them from time to time, or until the tofu is thoroughly cooked and browned.
- Make sure the outside of the tofu is somewhat crispy and golden brown.

Chicken and Broccoli Stir-Fry

Ingredients:
- One pound of thinly sliced, skinless, boneless chicken breasts
- Three cups of broccoli florets
- Two tsp soy sauce
- One spoonful of sauce made from oysters
- One tablespoon each of cornstarch, water, and spilt vegetable oil
- Two minced garlic cloves
- One teaspoon grated ginger
- One teaspoon of oil sesame
- Optional sesame seeds as a garnish
- Ready-to-serve cooked whole wheat noodles or brown rice

Instructions:
- Combine soy sauce, oyster sauce, cornstarch, and water in a small basin. Put aside.
- Combine 1 tablespoon of soy sauce with sliced chicken in a bowl. Give it 10 to 15 minutes to marinate.
- Heat up 1 tablespoon of vegetable oil over medium-high heat.
- Stir-fry the marinated chicken until it is cooked through and begins to take on some color.
- Bring out the chicken from the pan and set aside.
- Add one more tablespoon of oil to the same pan. Add the grated ginger and minced garlic. Stir-fry the broccoli florets for two to three minutes, or until they are crisp-tender.

- Add the cooked chicken and broccoli back to the pan. Cover the chicken and broccoli with the prepared sauce. Mix everything together until the chicken and broccoli are coated with a rich sauce.
- Pour some sesame oil onto the stir-fry and mix thoroughly. Garnish with sesame seeds, if desired.

Lean Beef and Vegetable Stir-Fry

Ingredients:
- One pound of thinly sliced lean beef, such as flank steak or sirloin
- Two teaspoons of low-sodium soy sauce
- One spoonful of sauce made from oysters
- One spoonful of sauce hoisin
- One tablespoon each of cornstarch and water
- Two tablespoons, split between two
- Two minced garlic cloves
- One teaspoon grated ginger
– One cup florets of broccoli
- One bell pepper, cut thinly
- One carrot (julienned)
- One cup (trimmed) snap peas
- One cup of sliced mushrooms
- Chopped green onions as a garnish
- Optional sesame seeds as a garnish
- Prepared cooked quinoa or brown rice for serving

Instructions:
- Mix the soy sauce, oyster sauce, hoisin sauce, cornstarch, and water in a small bowl. Put aside.

- Combine 1 tablespoon of soy sauce with the thinly sliced meat in a bowl. Give it 10 to 15 minutes to marinate.
- In a wok or big skillet over medium-high heat, heat 1 tablespoon of vegetable oil. When the beef is well cooked and browned, add the marinated steak and stir-fry. Take out the steak and place it aside.
- If necessary, add an additional tablespoon of oil to the same pan. Add the grated ginger and minced garlic. Add the snap peas, carrot, bell pepper, broccoli, and mushrooms. The veggies should be crisp-tender after three to five minutes of stir-frying.
- Add the stir-fried veggies and cooked beef back to the pan. Cover the beef and vegetables with the prepared sauce. Mix everything together until the steak and veggies are coated in a rich sauce.
- If preferred, garnish with sesame seeds and chopped green onions.

Cauliflower Fried Rice with Shrimp

Ingredients:
-One pound of peeled and deveined shrimp
- One medium head of grated or rice-like cauliflower
- Two teaspoons of soy sauce reduced in sodium
- One spoonful of sauce made from oysters
- One tablespoon each of sesame oil and vegetable oil
- Two beaten eggs
- One cup of mixed veggies (corn, carrots, and peas)

- Two minced garlic cloves
- One teaspoon grated ginger
- Three sliced green onions
- Salt and pepper to taste
- Fresh cilantro for decoration (optional)
- To serve, lime wedges

Instructions:
- Sprinkle salt and pepper on shrimp. Cook shrimp in a pan until they become opaque and pink. Put aside.
- Grate or pulse the cauliflower until it resembles rice.
- Combine oyster sauce, sesame oil, and soy sauce in a small bowl. Put aside.
- Heat vegetable oil in a large wok or skillet over medium-high heat. Add the grated ginger and minced garlic. Once the mixed vegetables are soft, stir them in.
- Add the grated cauliflower after pushing the vegetables to the side of the pan. Stir-fry the cauliflower for three to four minutes, or until it's cooked through but still somewhat crunchy.

- Add Shrimp and Sauce, Cover the shrimp and cauliflower with the sauce. Mix - Make a well in the middle and push the cauliflower mixture to the sides of the pan. Fill the well with the beaten eggs
- After letting the eggs settle for a little while, scramble them until they are thoroughly cooked.

- Stir the cauliflower mixture into the scrambled eggs. Add the finely chopped green onions. If needed, adjust the seasoning by tasting it.

Mushroom and Spinach Stuffed Chicken Breast

Ingredients:
- Four skinless and boneless chicken breasts
- One cup finely chopped mushrooms
- Two cups chopped fresh spinach
- Two minced garlic cloves
- One tablespoon olive oil
- Half cup crumbled low-fat feta cheese
- One teaspoon dried oregano
- Lemon wedges for serving
- Kitchen twine or toothpicks for tying
- Salt and pepper to taste

Instructions:
- Heat olive oil in a pan over medium heat. Add the chopped mushrooms and minced garlic. Sauté the mushrooms until they give off moisture and soften. Cook the chopped spinach until it wilts. Add salt, pepper, and dried oregano for seasoning. Take it off the fire and let it cool a little.
- Arrange every chicken breast evenly on a chopping block. Make a horizontal incision along the side of the breast with a sharp knife, being careful not to cut all the way through. Open the breast like a book to butterfly it.

- Spoon one side of each butterflied chicken breast with the mushroom and spinach mixture. Top the filling with crumble feta cheese
- Fold the other half of the chicken breast carefully over the filling and secure with toothpicks or twine. To keep the filling within, fasten the edges using toothpicks or kitchen thread.
- Sprinkle some salt, pepper, and dried oregano over the packed chicken breasts.
- Set the oven's temperature to 375°F, or 190°C. Arrange the stuffed chicken breasts onto a parchment paper-lined baking sheet. Bake the chicken for 25 to 30 minutes, or until the juices run clear and the chicken is cooked through.
- Make sure the chicken's internal temperature reaches 165°F (74°C).

Quinoa-Stuffed Bell Peppers

Ingredients:
- Four huge bell peppers cut in half and seeded
- One cup of rinsed quinoa
- Two cups water or veggie broth
- One tablespoon olive oil
- One finely sliced onion
- Two minced garlic cloves
- One chopped zucchini
- One cup of halved cherry tomatoes
One cup of rinsed and drained black beans
- One teaspoon each of chili powder and ground cumin

- One cup of shredded cheese (cherry, mozzarella, or any other type you choose) - Salt and pepper to taste
- Optional fresh parsley or cilantro garnish
- To serve, lime wedges

Instructions:
- Set the oven's temperature to 375°F, or 190°C.
- Halve the bell peppers and take out the seeds and membranes. The pepper halves should be put on a baking dish.
- Quinoa should be combined with vegetable broth (or water) in a saucepan. Bring to a boil, then lower heat, cover, and simmer until the quinoa is tender and the water has been absorbed, about 15 minutes.
- Heat the olive oil in a big skillet over medium heat. Put the chopped onion and garlic, and cook until they become very soft. Add the black beans, cherry tomatoes, and sliced zucchini. After 5 to 7 more minutes of cooking, the vegetables should be soft.
- Season the vegetable combination with salt, pepper, chili powder, and powdered cumin. Add the cooked quinoa and thoroughly combine.
- Stuff the quinoa and veggie mixture into each half of a bell pepper. Slightly press the filling down. Spread shredded cheese on top of each pepper.
- Bake the peppers for 25 to 30 minutes, or until they are soft, in a preheated oven, covered with aluminum foil.
- Make sure the cheese is melted and bubbling and the peppers are cooked to your preference.

Grilled Salmon with Quinoa and Roasted Vegetables

Ingredients:
- Two teaspoons olive oil
- Four salmon filets
- Two minced garlic cloves
- Two tablespoons of lemon juice
- One teaspoon of lemon zest
- Season with salt and pepper
- Garnish with fresh dill, if desired

Regarding Quinoa:
- One cup of washed quinoa
- Two cups water or veggie broth
- To taste salt

Roasted Vegetables
- 2 cups chopped mixed veggies (such as bell peppers, cherry tomatoes, zucchini, and asparagus).
- One tablespoon of olive oil
- One teaspoon dried thyme
- Salt and pepper to taste

Instructions:
- Olive oil, minced garlic, lemon zest, lemon juice, salt, and pepper should all be combined in a bowl. Apply the marinade to the salmon filets and let them sit for at least fifteen minutes.
- Turn the heat up to medium-high on your grill.

- Cook the salmon filets on the grill for 4–5 minutes
on each side, or until they are cooked through and
readily flake. Based on the thickness of the filets,
adjust cooking time.
- Quinoa should be combined with vegetable broth
(or water) in a saucepan. Bring to a boil, then lower
heat, cover, and simmer until the quinoa is tender
and the water has been absorbed, about 15
minutes. Add salt to taste and season.
- Set oven temperature to 400°F, or 200°C. Add
salt, pepper, dried thyme, and olive oil to the mixed
veggies and toss. Bake the veggies for 15 to 20
minutes, or until they are soft.

Vegetarian Stir-Fry with Tofu

Ingredients:
- Two tablespoons low-sodium soy sauce
- One tablespoon sesame oil
- One tablespoon cornstarch
- Two tablespoons split vegetable oil
- One finely sliced onion
- Two thinly sliced bell peppers (varying hues)
- One chopped carrot
- One cup of broccoli florets
- Two minced garlic cloves
- One tablespoon of grated ginger and two
teaspoons of hoisin sauce
- One tablespoon rice vinegar
- One tablespoon honey or maple syrup
- One tablespoon of optional sesame seeds as a
garnish

- Cooked brown rice or quinoa to serve
- Chopped green scallions for garnish

Instructions:
- Tofu should be pressed to eliminate extra water. Cut into cubes, then combine cornstarch, sesame oil, and soy sauce. Give it 15 to 20 minutes to marinate.
- Heat one tablespoon of vegetable oil in a big skillet or wok over medium-high heat. When golden brown on all sides, add the marinated tofu cubes and continue cooking. Take out the tofu and place it aside.
- Add one more tablespoon of vegetable oil to the same pan. Add the bell peppers, broccoli florets, sliced onion, and julienned carrot. Sauté the veggies for five to seven minutes, or until they are crisp-tender.
- Combine the vegetables with grated ginger and minced garlic. Stir-fry until aromatic, about one or two more minutes.
- Add the cooked tofu back to the pan along with the veggies. Combine the rice vinegar, hoisin sauce, and maple syrup (or honey) in a small bowl. Drizzle the tofu and veggies with the sauce. Mix everything until thoroughly coated.
- Add chopped green onions and sesame seeds to the vegetarian stir-fry with tofu.

CONCLUSION

For those who have just received a prostate cancer diagnosis, the prostate cancer diet cookbook offers a thorough roadmap for managing the dietary complications during a trying period. It is more than just a cookbook; it becomes a helpful ally, offering vital information about selecting a diet that is specifically suited to the requirements of people with prostate cancer.
This cookbook aims to empower people on their path to better health by carefully considering nutritional research and culinary experience. Prostate-friendly components and well-considered recipe choices are combined to produce a beneficial effect on general health.

The cookbook explores the nuances of how particular nutrients may affect prostate health, going beyond taste and flavor. It acts as a lighthouse of information, guiding people to understand the mutually beneficial relationship between diet and the body's defense against cancer. Through the dissemination of knowledge regarding the functions of antioxidants, foods high in anti-inflammatory compounds, and other essential components, the cookbook helps to initiate preventive health care.

It provides flexible recipes that may be adjusted to accommodate different appetites and dietary needs that may develop throughout treatment. This flexibility guarantees that the cookbook will continue to be a useful and trustworthy resource for the duration of the patient's therapy.

In the end, the newly diagnosed patient's prostate cancer diet cookbook proves to be a comprehensive resource that promotes wellbeing and a sense of control. It is evidence of the revolutionary potential of diet when combined with conventional medical procedures. The cookbook turns into a reliable ally as people set out on this journey of health and culinary exploration, enabling them to make decisions that support a strong and well-fed body.